Work-related Musculoskeletal Disorders

Edited by Orhan Korhan

Published in London, United Kingdom

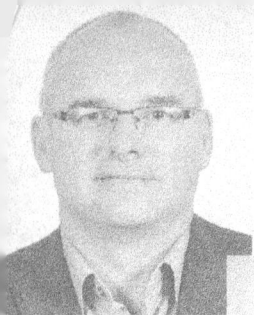
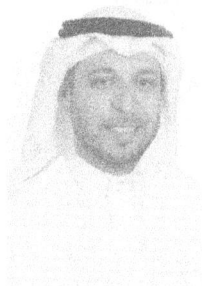
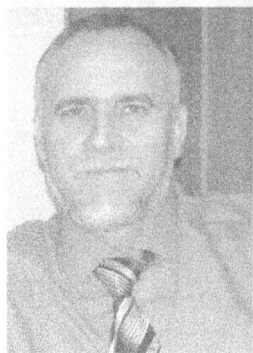
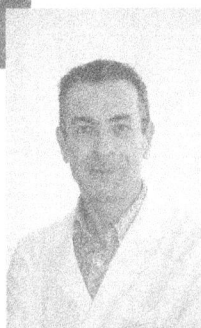
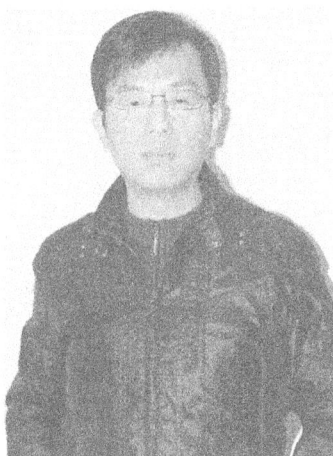
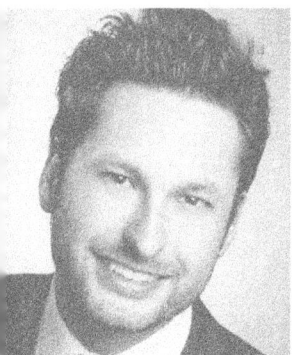
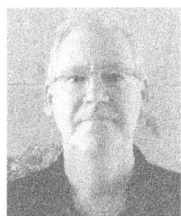

IntechOpen

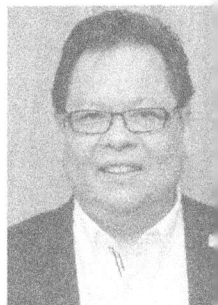
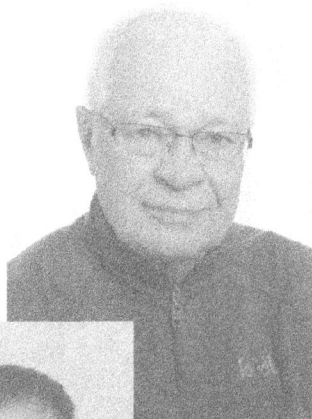
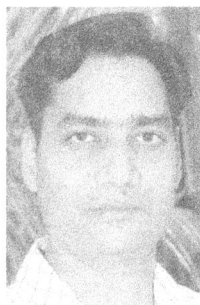
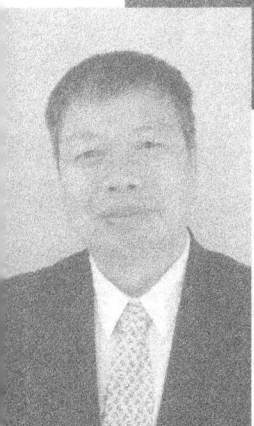
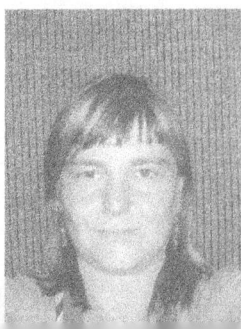
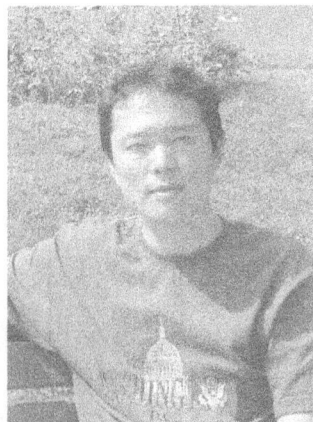

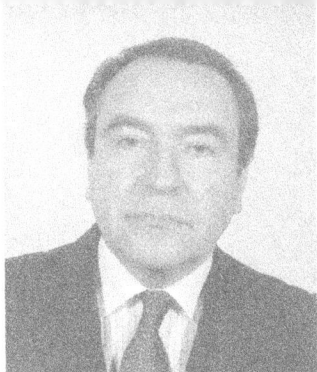

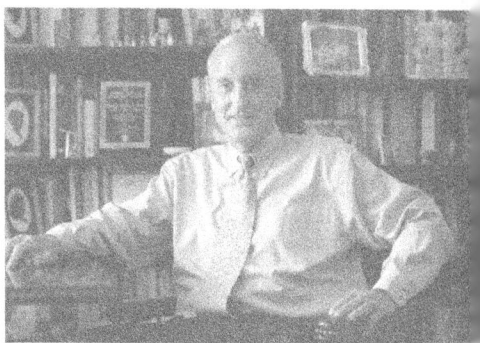

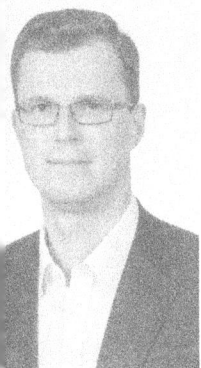

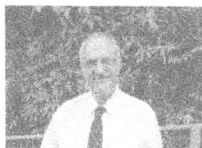

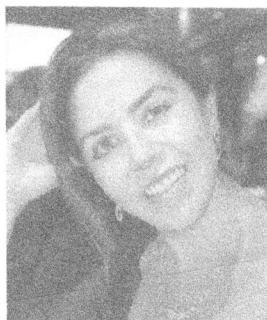

Supporting open minds since 2005

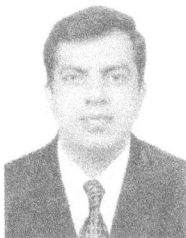

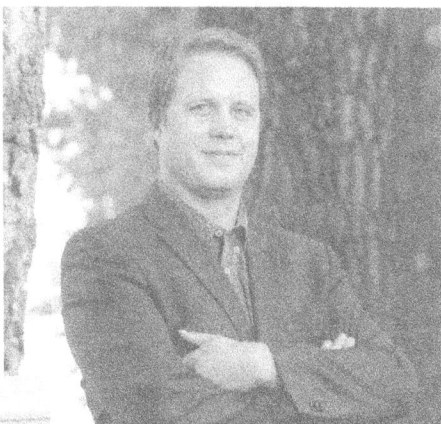

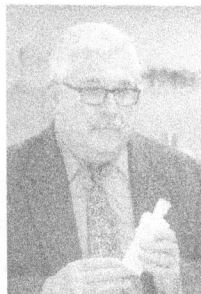

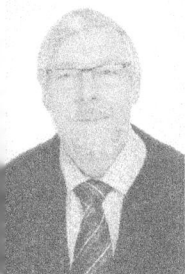

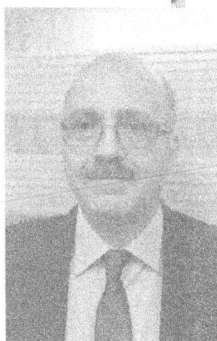

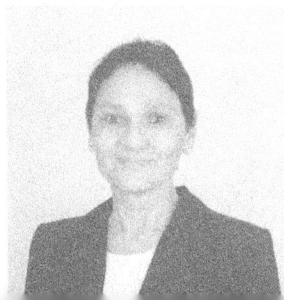

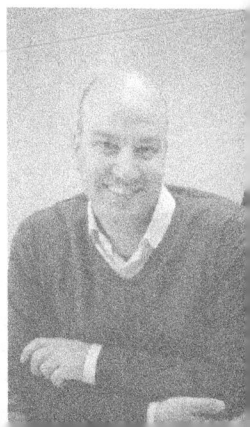

Work-related Musculoskeletal Disorders
http://dx.doi.org/10.5772/intechopen.78458
Edited by Orhan Korhan

Contributors
Martha Roselia Contreras-Valenzuela, Roy Lopez-Sesenes, Alber Eduardo Duque Alvarez, Alejandro David Guzmán-Clemente, Viridiana Aydee Leòn Hernandez, Francisco Cuenca-Jiménez, Francisco Cuenca-Jimenez, Yusuf Erdem, Jenson Mak, Orhan Korhan

Notice
Statements and opinions expressed in the chapters are these of the individual contributors and not necessarily those of the editors or publisher. No responsibility is accepted for the accuracy of information contained in the published chapters. The publisher assumes no responsibility for any damage or injury to persons or property arising out of the use of any materials, instructions, methods or ideas contained in the book.

First published in London, United Kingdom, 2019 by IntechOpen
IntechOpen is the global imprint of INTECHOPEN LIMITED, registered in England and Wales, registration number: 11086078, The Shard, 25th floor, 32 London Bridge Street London, SE19SG – United Kingdom
Printed in Croatia

British Library Cataloguing-in-Publication Data
A catalogue record for this book is available from the British Library

Additional hard and PDF copies can be obtained from orders@intechopen.com

Work-related Musculoskeletal Disorders
Edited by Orhan Korhan
p. cm.
Print ISBN 978-1-78985-234-9
Online ISBN 978-1-78985-695-8
eBook (PDF) ISBN 978-1-78985-696-5

We are IntechOpen,
the world's leading publisher of
Open Access books
Built by scientists, for scientists

4,300+
Open access books available

116,000+
International authors and editors

130M+
Downloads

Our authors are among the

151
Countries delivered to

Top 1%
most cited scientists

12.2%
Contributors from top 500 universities

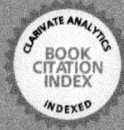

Interested in publishing with us?
Contact book.department@intechopen.com

Numbers displayed above are based on latest data collected.
For more information visit www.intechopen.com

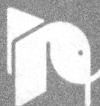

Meet the editor

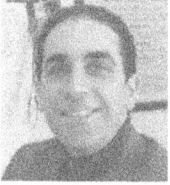

Orhan Korhan obtained a BS from Eastern Mediterranean University, Northern Cyprus, in 2000, a MS from the University of Louisville, Kentucky, in 2002, and a PhD in Industrial Engineering from Eastern Mediterranean University in 2010. He has been working at Eastern Mediterranean University since 2009. He became Assistant Professor in 2010 and Associate Professor in 2014. He is a board member of the Continuous Education Center and is currently Academic Affairs Coordinator at the Rector's Office. He has been assigned to the scientific committees of several international conferences and has published several books, book chapters, and papers in various countries. His current research interests include work-related musculoskeletal disorders, cognitive ergonomics, educational ergonomics, human–computer interaction, Industry 4.0, and facilities planning and design.

Contents

Preface

Musculoskeletal disorders (MSDs) are injuries that affect the musculoskeletal system of the human body, especially bones, spinal discs, tendons, joints, ligaments, cartilage, nerves, and blood vessels.

Work-related musculoskeletal disorders (WRMSDs) are often observed when there is a discrepancy between the physical capacity of the human body and the physical requirements of the work task. Along with personal factors such as personal medical history, the design of the physical and psychosocial working environment can contribute to the formation of these disorders.

This book describes the human musculoskeletal system, including such topics as anthropometry and posture, as it relates to accidents and injuries in the workplace. Chapters discuss such subjects as job standards; risk assessment; direct and indirect costs of WRMSDs; epidemiology, etiology, and pathology of WRMSDs; engineering and administrative controls; risk factor identification; injury management; and education and training. It presents a holistic approach to identifying, intervening, and preventing WRMSDs.

Orhan Korhan
Eastern Mediterranean University,
Famagusta, North Cyprus, Turkey

Section 1

Definiton of WRMSDs

Chapter 1

Introductory Chapter: Work-Related Musculoskeletal Disorders

Orhan Korhan and Asad Ahmed Memon

1. Introduction

According to the National Institute for Occupational Safety and Health [1], musculoskeletal disorder (MSD) is a damage that affects the musculoskeletal system of the human body, especially at bones, spinal discs, tendons, joints, ligaments, cartilage, nerves, and blood vessels. Such injuries may result due to repetitive motions, forces, and vibrations on human bodies during executing certain job activities. Previous injuries, physical condition, heredity, pregnancy, lifestyle, and poor diet are the factors that contribute to the musculoskeletal symptoms.

Work-related musculoskeletal symptoms can be observed at workplaces when there is a discrepancy between the physical capacity of the human body and the physical requirements of the task. Musculoskeletal disorders can be related to the work activities and conditions, and they could significantly contribute to the development of MSDs. However, these are not necessarily the only causes or significant risk factors.

The World Health Organization recognizes conditions that result in pain and functional impairment that affect the neck, shoulders, elbows, forearms, wrists, and hands as work related when the work activities and work conditions significantly contribute to the development of work-related disorders (**Figure 1**).

Work-related musculoskeletal disorders (WRMSDs) are described as wide range of degenerative and inflammatory conditions that affect the supporting blood vessels, peripheral nerves, joints, ligaments, tendons, and muscles. Such conditions could result in functional impairment and pain which are widely experienced at the upper extremities and the neck [2].

At the workplace, the causes of musculoskeletal disorders are diverse but poorly understood. Aptel et al. [3] stated that biomechanical factors such as repetitive motion, strenuous efforts, extreme joint postures, and/or psychosocial factors establish the key role in work-related musculoskeletal disorders. In [4], it is provided that certain psychological factors are associated with musculoskeletal discomfort and may eventually provide one way to intervene to reduce MSDs.

This chapter aims to analyze the ergonomics, administration of occupational health and safety, economic impact, prevalence, intervention, and prevention of WRMSDs.

2. Risk factors

Hales and Bernard [5] cited the causes of work-related musculoskeletal symptoms in two categories: physical and psychosocial.

PERSON	WORKPLACE
Demographic Structure • Genetic Factors • Anthropometric Characteristics • Individual Factors **Symptoms** • Biomechanic Strain • Fatigue • Discomort **Frequency of Symptoms** **Personal Medical History**	**Physical Work Environment** • Equipment/Device use • Works tasks • Internal Loads • Psychological Response • Duration of Work **Psychosocial Work Environment** • External Loads • Organizational Factors • Social Support • Psychological Profile Workstation Design

WORK-RELATED MUSCULOSKELETAL DISORDERS

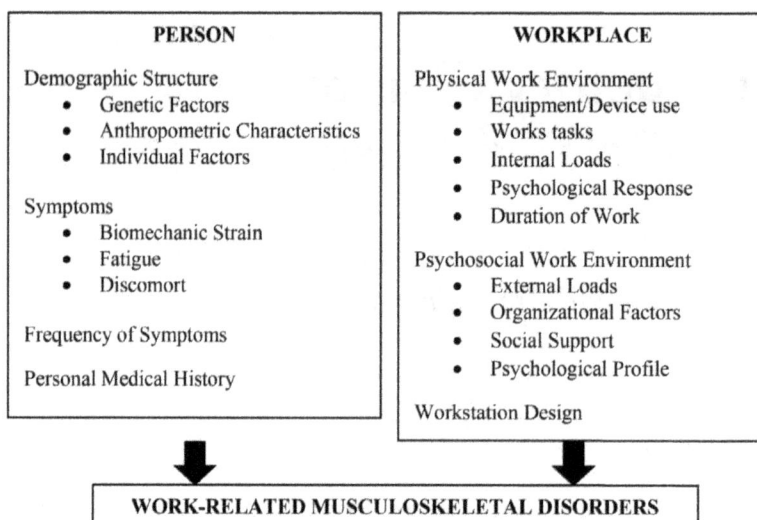

Figure 1.
Factors scheme.

2.1 Physical factors

These include intense, repeated, or sustained exertions; awkward, non-neutral, and extreme postures; rapid work pace; repeated and/or prolonged activity; insufficient time for recovery, vibration, and cold temperatures.

2.1.1 Inappropriate postures

The muscles and joints involved in an activity and the amount of stress or force tolerated or generated are determined by the body posture due to the fact that as the back bends, there is more stress exerted on the spinal discs during object lifting, handling, or lowering than when the back is straight. The tasks requiring sustained or repeated twisting or bending of the shoulders, wrists, hips, and the knees also increase the stress on the joints. Therefore, prolonged or frequent work activities can be very stressful.

2.1.2 Repetitive motions

Frequently repeated motions (e.g., every few seconds) and prolonged periods could end up in accumulated muscle-tendon strain and fatigue. If the time allocated between the exertions is sufficient, the muscles and tendons can recover from forceful exertions and stretching effects. During inappropriate postures and forceful exertions, the impact of repetitive motions due to performing the same work activities can be increased. Risk factor such as repetitive actions can also depend of the performed specific act and the body area.

2.1.3 Duration

The amount of time that someone is continuously exposed to a risk factor is called duration. The job tasks that require the use of the same motions or muscles for long periods increase the probability of general and local fatigue. Generally, if the period of the continuous work increases (for the tasks require extended muscle contraction), more rest or recovery period is required.

2.1.4 Frequency

Within a given period of time, the number of repeated exertions by a person is defined as frequency. In fact, if the exertion is repeated more often, the speed of movement of the exerted body part increases. Moreover, the recovery period decreases when more frequent exertion is completed, and this increases the probability of general and local fatigue with the duration.

2.2 Psychosocial factors

WRMSDs do not only result in the physical stressors. However, a set of multiple factors determine the formation. Psychosocial risk factors such as stressful job, social pressure at work, and job dissatisfaction are such factors which contribute to the formation of WRMSDs. When an injury occurs, psychosocial factors, such as incongruous pain and depression, are the main reasons for the development of a disability and transition from acute to chronic pain [6].

These include monotonous work, time pressure, a high workload, unorganized work-rest schedules, complexity of tasks, career concerns, lack of peer support, a poor relationship between workers and their supervisors, and poor organizational characteristics (climate, culture, and communications).

The way to structure and manage the work processes are called as organization of work and it deals with the following subjects:

- Work scheduling (work-rest schedules, work hours, and shift work).

- Job design (task complexity, required effort and skill, and the degree of control of work).

- Interpersonal facets of work (relationships with colleagues, subordinates, and supervisors).

- Concerns regarding career (job security and opportunities to grow).

- Style of management (teamwork and participatory management).

- Characteristics of the organization (culture, communication, and climate).

Many of the above components are called as "psychosocial factors," and they are known as risk factors for psychological strain and job stress. Stress is a conceived emotional and physical reaction of the human body to events or circumstances which cause excitement, danger, confusion, irritation, or frightening. Particularly, it is a transition from someone's normal behavior according to a cause that results in tear and wear on the body's mental or physical resources.

There are internal or external stimuli that cause stress. The internal stimuli are those stressors that involve self-expectations, impersonal barriers, and conflicting desires. Apparently, internal stimuli depend on personal aspects. However, external stimuli include situations where expectations, time limit, lack of resources, and lack of vision and goals present.

Stressors may be physiological, psychological, social, environmental, developmental, spiritual, or cultural and represent unmet needs. Stress causes changes in the human body that are usually centered on the nervous system and endocrine system. Therefore, the human body's internal environment is constantly changing, and the body's adaptive mechanisms continually function to adjustments in heart rate, respiratory rate, blood pressure, temperature, fluid and electrolyte balances, hormone secretions, and level of consciousness.

Intensive and extensive stress results in disorders in the musculoskeletal system. Emotions like anger, frustration, irritation, confusion, tension, and nervousness cause the stress. It is not only the experience and frequency of such feelings but also the repetition of the activities and motions that induce injuries or musculoskeletal disorders.

In considering human emotions and feelings and applying the results of the research to their impact on the musculoskeletal system, it is probably platitudinous to make a statement that the greater the knowledge and understanding of the human being, the better the result obtained. In order to identify and understand the effect of the emotions on the musculoskeletal system, important risk factors for musculoskeletal disorders should be recognized.

2.3 Psychological risk factors

Moreover, together with the above conditions, some other work aspects contribute to both physical and psychological stress as well. The human body in fact is limited in kinematic motions as it is a mechanism formed by biological characteristics. Beyond this, it also includes a brain which thinks, reasons, and feels. Thus, feelings such as joy, pain, anger, sadness, depression, frustration, outrage, boredom, fear, jealousy, hate, love, and (even) schizophrenia are experienced by human beings.

When exposed to stress, human beings show responses such as fear, frustration, anger, fatigue, tension, depression, anxiety, helplessness, confusion, and lack of vigor.

3. Common types of occupational MSDs

i. Tendonitis: it is the most common hand problem, which happens when the tendons connecting the fingers to muscles in the forearms get inflamed. Tendons help attach muscle to bone to allow movement of a joint [7].

ii. Tenosynovitis: this is another common ailment, where the synovial sheaths (sacks filled with fluid) swell which surround and protect the tendons. Carpal tunnel syndrome (CTS) is the condition which is a result of this swelling. The carpal tunnel is a small opening close to the bottom of the hand which accommodates the tendons and the median nerve that provides sensation to the hand. In the case of swelling of the synovial sheaths, the carpal tunnel cramps and puts pressure on the nerve. There are several syndromes of the CTS, but the most frequent ones are numbness, tingling, or a burning sensation in the palms, fingers, and wrists. These conditions can lead to strength and sensation loss in the hands in time [7].

iii. Nerve compression: throughout the body, there are several nerves that transmit signals from the body parts to the brain. These often move in the spine through small tunnels available between the vertebrae. There are many conditions which cause the nerves to become compressed, pinched, or squeezed, which can result in weakness, numbness, severe pain, and loss of coordination. The condition in which the sciatic nerve in the spine becomes compressed is known as sciatica. The symptoms of this condition appear in the back of the leg and at the side of the foot [7].

iv. Raynaud's syndrome/disease: this is a loss of blood circulation, which results in whitening and numbness of the finders. It is sometimes called "white finger," "wax finger," or "dead finger" [7].

v. Reflex sympathetic dystrophy: this is a rare, incurable condition character-ized by fry, swollen hands and loss of muscle control. It is consistently painful [7].

vi. Ganglion cyst: this disorder arise when a swelling or lump in the wrist result-ing from jelly-like substance leaks from a joint or tendon sheath [7].

vii. Cervical radiculopathy: this is the condition of an injury due to the extend-ing out of those nerves that provide sensation and trigger movement from cervical vertebrae which result in weakness, numbness, or pain in the hand, wrist, arm, or shoulder [7].

viii. Lateral epicondylitis: this is a condition when the outer part of the elbow becomes painful and tender, usually as a result of a specific strain, overuse, or a direct bang [7].

ix. Rheumatoid arthritis: this is a disabling autoimmune disease which is progressive and happens in a long term. It causes pain, swelling, and inflam-mation in and around the joints and other body organs. Hands and feet are affected mainly, but it can be seen in any joint as well. It usually occurs at the same joints on both sides of the body [7].

4. Economic impact

Musculoskeletal disorders (MSD) are a major concern globally not just due to the pain and disability suffered by the individual worker but also due to its economic impact not just on the employer but also on the society as a whole. In 2013/2014, 8.3 million work days were lost in UK due to musculoskeletal disorders [8]. In the European Union (EU), more than 40 million workers are affected by musculoskel-etal disorders that translate to one in seven people [9]. In the USA, musculoskeletal disorders accounted for 29–35% of the occupational injuries in private industries which resulted in absence from work from 1992 to 2010 [10].

Financial costs due to musculoskeletal disorders can be divided into direct costs and indirect costs. Direct costs are the costs mainly comprised of medical expen-ditures which are used to cure and/or prevent diseases. These include resources such as hospitals, doctors, equipment, etc. Indirect costs are the hidden costs which include costs due to loss of productivity, training, and hiring costs of new employ-ees. These productivity losses occur when either the person is sick and does not show up at work or his productivity is reduced while at work due to sickness. There is also cost due to loss of unpaid work due to sickness when the person is not able to do his household tasks.

In both manufacturing and service sector, productivity loss is one of the big-gest and severe problems. Organizations suffer from decreased job productivity and employee absence which then creates significant economic burden not just for them but for the economy as a whole. Despite significant indirect costs due to musculoskeletal disorders, many economic evaluations done by countries exclude these costs which are greater than the direct costs. Even the countries which do include these costs significantly vary in their methodology from one another due to disagreement over the current methods and the certain flaws in them.

Ignoring or including only some part of these costs in economic evaluations has a twofold effect: firstly, health benefits as a result of a proposed health intervention are underestimated and, secondly, not enough resources are allocated to research in workplace safety and health as a result of under estimation of these costs. In the USA, despite occupational injuries costing society up to $250 billion, a budget of $0.3 billion was allocated to the National Institute of Occupational Safety and Health (NIOSH) in 2013 [11]. This compared with budget of $5 billion for National Cancer Institute which costs society up to $219 billion.

For businesses to remain competitive, it is important that research of safe workplace practices is promoted and the businesses are given guidance about workplace safety because without a healthy human resource, no entity can grow. This can only happen when these costs are captured in economic evaluations and given their due attention by both the employer and the society as a whole.

4.1 Costs of MSDs

Calculation of costs of MSDs is not straightforward as several factors need to be considered before total costs are computed. The following components need to be estimated to calculate the total costs of MSDs [12].

i. Direct costs: these are the costs spent on management of musculoskeletal disorders, i.e., medical costs, administrative, compensation, and insurance costs. These costs are visible, and estimation of these is straightforward. These costs are not within the scope of this chapter and thus would not be discussed further.

ii. Indirect costs: these are hidden costs which include costs for lost productivity both paid and unpaid, lost earnings and tax revenues, lost opportunity costs for careers, and costs of hiring and training new workers. These costs are difficult to estimate, and in the literature, most of the debate is around calculation of these costs. This will be discussed later in detail.

iii. Intangible costs: this includes psychosocial burden such as job stress, family stress, and economic stress which leads to reduced quality of life [12]. As these costs are very difficult to express in monetary terms, they are rarely considered for cost calculations. But intangible costs give useful information about the quality of life of people with MSDs and help in measuring effectiveness of the interventions. Intangible costs are usually expressed with the help of a measure called quality adjusted life years (QALY). Even though these costs are not the focus of this study, they have been mentioned in the context of explaining methods of measuring indirect costs.

4.2 National data of costs due to MSDs

Coyte et al. [13] estimated that the total cost of musculoskeletal costs in Canada in 1994 was $25.6 billion (Canadian) which equates to 3.4% GDP of Canada.

Indirect costs were 2.4 times of the direct costs. Lost productivity cost due to disability was $13.9 billion dollars which is 54.3% of the total cost.

The French Government in a press release part of national Plan on Health & Safety at Work (Plain Sante Travail 2005–2009) highlighted that 75% of all the occupational diseases in 2005 were musculoskeletal disorders [14]. Thirty-one thousand diseases were compensated which lead to loss of 6.5 million work days and 650 million EUR. Indirect costs are not included in this amount.

In the UK, 8.3 million days were lost due to MSDs in 2013/2014, which equates to 15.9 days per case of MSDs [8]. It cost around £4.5 billion in lost productivity to Britain due to work-related illnesses in 2012/2013 [15]. The direct cost of MSD in Korea is estimated as $4.5 billion, whereas cost due to loss of productivity is $2.28 billion [16]. The total economic cost was estimated to be $6.89 billion, which amounts to 0.7% of the GDP.

In the USA, the economic cost of MSDs is estimated between $45 and 54 billion [17]. These include costs such as compensation costs, lost productivity, and lost wages. In the USA, work-related musculoskeletal disorders (WRMSD) account for 34% lost workdays; direct costs for worker compensations are estimated to be $20 billion, whereas indirect costs can be five times more than the direct costs [18].

Data which is available in a German national report on safety and health estimated that 95 million days are lost due to MSD which costs €23.9 [14]. Wenig et al. [19] calculated the total costs for back pain for Germany. The study indicated a cost of around 49 billion EUR. Average back pain costs were around 1300 EUR per patient per year. 46% of the total comprised of direct costs and 54% comprised of indirect costs.

Deloitte Access Economics calculated the indirect costs for people with arthritis and other musculoskeletal conditions to be $11.2 billion in Australia in 2012 [20]. This amount is 55% of the total health cost. Out of this amount, productivity costs accounted for $7.4 billion, which included costs associated with reduced employment ($6 billion), lost superannuation, absenteeism, and presenteeism.

In a French study commissioned by the national working conditions agency (ANACT) to estimate cost of MSDs in three companies with more than 500 employees, it was found that indirect costs were 10–30 times higher than direct costs [14]. Total cost was between €6800 and €11,200 per employee.

5. Intervention and prevention

The European Agency for Safety and Health at Work (2008) suggested that it is possible to draw the following conclusions about the different types of interventions based on the randomized and non-randomized comparative studies in the workplace, trials without a comparison group, and laboratory studies:

- Organizational and administrative interventions. Only a few studies were conducted on these type of interventions. In physically demanding works, the evidence is limited to show that the disorders at the neck and shoulder regions can be reduced when there is a reduction in daily work hours (from 7 to 6 hours). Also, it has been shown that without productivity loss, it is possible to introduce extra breaks within repetitive work. However, the methods to be applied prevent the occurrence of MSDs effectively are not clear and yet requires to be studied.

- Technical, engineering, or ergonomic interventions. The workload on the back without any productivity loss can be reduced by applying certain technical measures. Very few evidence is available to illustrate that these measures can reduce absenteeism due to illness and low back disorders. However, there is strong evidence to show that the load on the shoulders, arms, and hands can be reduced by ergonomic hand tools. Moreover, literature is limited to illustrate the reduction of MSDs due to manual computer tasks or vibration.

- Protective equipment. It is not clear whether the use of back belts helps or hurts the back pain. It could not be achieved scientifically that the use of back belt can prevent back pain during manual material handling. Also, there is no evidence on prevention of upper limb disorders by using other protective equipment.

- Behavioral modification. It is widely discussed in the literature that training on work methods is not adequate if it is used as the sole measure to prevent the back pain. Reduction in the relapses of shoulder-neck pain and back pain by physical training is another issue which yet requires to be studied extensively. Therefore, the training should involve dynamic exercises, which are to be repeated three times a week at least, in order to be effective.

6. Discussion and conclusion

Occupational injuries pose costly health problems (direct cost) and lost productivity (indirect cost) problems in workplaces where people are engaged in intensive, repetitive action and long hours of work. Direct costs occupy only 25% of the total induced cost of WRMSDs. Thus, ergonomic interventions in the workplace should be organized to focus on the reduction of the lost productivity, as it occupies the majority of the costs.

Alone or in a combination, the risk factors that contribute to the formation of WRMSDs can be physical, psychological, or psychosocial. Psychosocial and physical occupational risk factors should be analyzed in detail to understand the effect on the organization. Primarily, the working conditions should be analyzed for awkward postures and repetitive jobs.

WRMSDs may cause pain, slow responses, increased probabilities of accidents, reduced quality of life, and working ability. Therefore, both the individuals and the organizations should accept the fact that they are under a constant risk, and they should get ergonomic training in which they should apply at every step of their lives to be protected from WRMSDs.

Author details

Orhan Korhan[1]* and Asad Ahmed Memon[2]

1 Eastern Mediterranean University, Famagusta, North Cyprus, Turkey

2 Warwick Manufacturing Group, The University of Warwick, Coventry, UK

*Address all correspondence to: orhan.korhan@emu.edu.tr

IntechOpen

References

[1] National Institute for Occupational Safety and Health. Musculoskeletal Disorders and Workplace Factors. Columbia Parkway Cincinnati, OH: U.S. Department of Health and Human Services; 1997

[2] Korhan O, Mackieh A. A model for occupational injury risk assessment of musculoskeletal discomfort and their frequencies in computer users. Safety Science. 2010;**48**(7):868-877

[3] Aptel M, Aublet-Cuvelier A, Cnockaert JC. Work-Related Musculoskeletal Disorders of the Upper Limb. 2002;**69**:546-555

[4] Mekhora K, Liston CB, Nanthanvanij S, Cole JH. The effect of ergonomic intervention on discomfort in computer users with tension neck syndrome. International Journal of Industrial Ergonomics. 2000;**26**:367-379

[5] Hales TR, Bernard BP. Epidemiology of work-related musculoskeletal disorders. The Orthopedic Clinics of North America. 1996;**27**(4):679-709

[6] Menzel NN. Psychosocial factors in musculoskeletal disorders. Critical Care Nursing Clinics of North America. 2007;**19**(2):145-153

[7] OSHA Technical Manual (OTM). Information Date: 1/20/1999. Directive Number: TED 01-00-015 [TED 1-0.15A]. Constitution Avenue NW, Washington, DC; 1999

[8] Health and Safety Executive. Musculoskeletal disorders in Great Britain 2014. In: Health and Safety Executive. 2014b. http://www.hse.gov.uk/statistics/overall/hssh1415.pdf (visited on March 26, 2019)

[9] Bevan S et al. Fit for Work? Musculoskeletal Disorders in the European Workforce. London: The Work Foundation; 2009

[10] AFL-CIO. Death on the Job Report. AFL-CIO [Online]. 2013. Available from: https://aflcio.org/reports/death-job-2013 [accessed on March 26, 2019]

[11] Leigh JP. At $250B, Costs of Occupational Injury and Illness Exceed Costs of Cancer. Economic Policy Institute; 2013. https://www.epi.org/blog/250b-costs-occupational-injury-illness-exceed/ (posted January 3, 2013, visited on March 26, 2019)

[12] WHO Scientific Group. The Burden of Musculoskeletal Conditions at the Start of the New Millennium. Geneva: World Health Organisation; 2003

[13] Coyte PC, Asche CV, Croxford R, Chan B. The economic cost of musculoskeletal disorders in Canada. Arthritis & Rheumatology. 1998;**11**(5):315-325

[14] EU-OSHA. OSH in Figures: Work-Related Musculoskeletal Disorders in the EU—Facts and Figures. Luxembourg: Publications Office of the European Union; 2010

[15] Health and Safety Executive. Costs to Britain of workplace fatalities and self-reported injuries and ill health, 2012/13. In: Health and Safety Executive. 2014a

[16] Oh I-H et al. The economic burden of musculoskeletal disease in Korea: A cross sectional study. BMC Musculoskeletal Disorders. 2011;**12**(1):157

[17] National Research Council and Institute of Medicine. Musculoskeletal Disorders and the Workplace: Low Back and Upper Extremities. Washington, DC: The

National Academies Press; 2001. DOI:
10.17226/10032

[18] OSHA. 1218-AB58. Prevention
of Work-Related Musculoskeletal
Disorders. Constitution Avenue NW,
Washington, DC: Occupational Safety
and Health Administration; 2014

[19] Wenig CM et al. Costs of back pain
in Germany. European Journal of Pain.
2009;**13**(3):280-286

[20] Arthritis and Osteoporosis Victoria.
A Problem Worth Solving: The Rising
Cost of Musculoskeletal Conditions
in Australia. Elsternwick, Victoria:
Arthritis and Osteoporosis; 2013

Section 2

Prevalence of WRMSDs

A Methodology for Detecting Musculoskeletal Disorders in Industrial Workplaces Using a Mapping Representation of Risk

Martha Roselia Contreras-Valenzuela,
Alejandro David Guzmán-Clemente and
Francisco Cuenca-Jiménez

Abstract

A correct identification of ergonomic risks and their physical location in production areas becomes vital for the prevention of work-related illnesses. The method proposed for detecting musculoskeletal disorders (MSDs) in industrial workplaces has the objective of identifying the relationship between the workplace design and the nonergonomic task content. A mapping of work conditions was implemented to develop a diagnosis about hazards and ergonomic risk factors present in the work system. The information collected was organized in an ergonomic risk map with the following structure: inputs, information about risks and hazards, process, information about how the risk exposure leads to MSDs and outputs, and information about the consequences of risk factor exposure. The mapping results allowed determining the causes of work-related illnesses in activities of polishing and screening metals, establishing as a main cause of risk the barrel height (1.70 m) that forces the material handling above the shoulders. Force demands required to perform the task (around 277 N in each lifting) were determined. The work-related illnesses identified were low back injuries and rotator cuff injures. The information contained in the map improves the understanding of employers and workers about the origin of ergonomic problems and supports the decision-making about improvement projects focused on risk elimination.

Keywords: ergonomics, musculoskeletal disorders, process mapping, risk assessment, hazard identification

1. Introduction

The specialist designing workplaces, equipment, and tools and selecting workers for a specific task must understand the purpose of designing activities and devices that need muscular strengths. The human muscle strength measurement is important for understanding human capabilities. Nevertheless, the knowledge about strengths developed by an individual during work does not give the specialist enough information to solve ergonomic problems that lead to musculoskeletal disorders (MSDs). Thus, a work-system elements assessment should be necessary to find hazards that cause microtraumas [1]. The microtraumas outrun the body's recovery system causing work-related injuries that result in musculoskeletal disorders (MSDs).

From a mechanical point of view, when a machine repeats intensely specific movements during its operation, the applied forces cause fatigue in its mechanisms [2]. From a biomechanical point of view, the musculoskeletal system suffers from fatigue and wears down in joints and muscle injuries [3], when there are ergonomic risk factors at work such as employees' prolonged exposure time to awkward postures, excessive force exertion, repetitive movements, and manual material handling, causing fatigue and impacting on the health and well-being of workers [4, 5].

Consequently, a correct identification of ergonomic risks and their physical location in production areas becomes vital for the prevention of work-related illnesses.

1.1 Development of MSDs: Current situation in Mexico

In Mexico, MSDs were included in the work-related illness classification by the Mexican Health Secretary (SSA) until 2008. The Mexican Institute of Social Safety (known as IMSS) categorized the information about MSDs into seven diseases and one injury. This catalog is named "MSDs classification according to a kind of injury" and contains the following diseases [8]:

1. Other synovitis, tenosynovitis, and bursitis

2. Radial styloid tenosynovitis (Quervain)

3. Shoulder injury

4. Carpal tunnel syndrome

5. Epicondylitis

6. Other enthesopathies

7. Osteoarthritis/arthrosis

8. Dorsopathies

In 2009, the number of MSDs was recounted for the first time. **Table 1** presents data of a nine-year period (2009–2017) [6, 7]. During that period, the IMSS reported only 20,523 cases, showing an underreporting problem. Aspects like authorities not properly reporting risk conditions or workers' fear of being fired if they notify symptoms, as well as employers' evasion of mandatory law compliance [8, 9], contribute to the problem of lack of information. Despite work related-illnesses not being appropriately studied as MSDs yet, there was a data ascendant tendency in the results; see **Figure 1**.

In Mexico City, during the first forum on safety and health at work carried out in August 2015, it was determined that MSDs will be subjects of care because of their impact on workers' health [10]. To abate this health problem, the Mexican Ministry of Labour and Social Safety Secretaria del Trabajo y Previsión Social (STPS) issued a mandatory rule called Federal Rule for Safety and Health at Work (Reglamento Federal de Seguridad y Salud en el Trabajo) in November 2014 [11].

Year	Work-related illnesses	Work-related injuries	Percentage of MSDs with respect to work-related injuries
2009	266	4101	6.49
2010	513	3466	15.80
2011	788	4105	19.20
2012	1309	4853	26.97
2013	1893	6364	29.75
2014	2604	8301	31.37
2015	3722	12,009	30.99
2016	4273	12,622	33.85
2017	5155	14,159	36.41
Total	20,523	69,980	29.33

Table 1.
Total cases of MSDs developed by workers in Mexico reported by the IMSS [8, 9].

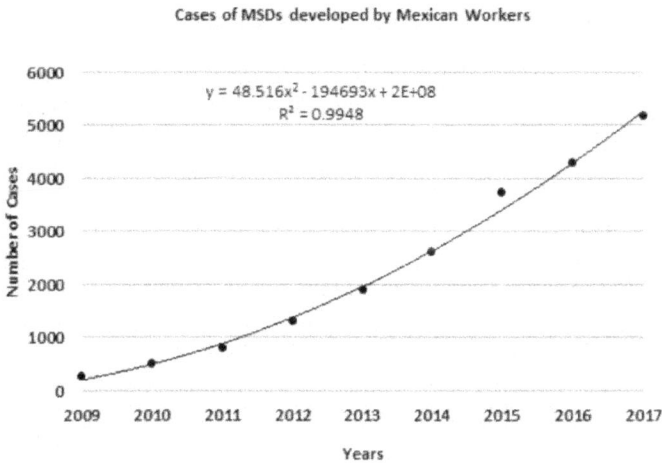

Figure 1.
Data ascendant tendency of MSD cases developed by workers in Mexico [8, 9].

It includes a new employer obligation for identifying, reporting, and reducing ergonomic risks inside facilities. Now, ergonomic risk factors are highlighted. Hence, the correct identification of MSDs becomes a big problem for the employers. Thus, the identification of ergonomic risk and musculoskeletal disorders (MSDs) for their prevention is too important. The aim of identifying the risks is to find process conditions that lead to musculoskeletal disorders and work-system elements that need changes from an ergonomic point of view.

In this chapter, a methodology for detecting musculoskeletal disorders was employed in a case study, and the diagnosis and analysis developed were used to propose a mapping representation of risks inside the workplace. The mapping resulted in a standardized representation of risks to ensure risk identification. The method includes (a) reports of the employees' complaints about workstation design and symptomatology suffered by workers as input information, (b) a description about the nonergonomic elements of the task and biomechanical studies on ergonomic risk factors that cause MSDs, (c) risk assessment results and work-related injuries and illnesses as output information, and (d) the cost of nonergonomics spent per year giving extra information that supports the decision-making about future ergonomic interventions and workstation redesign.

2. Mapping process tool

There are representations of conditions from an ergonomic point of view, for example, the empirical design of a human-machine system about the person-process relationship designed by Lemon [12], which involves an analysis about job organization, environment, and workplace; however, his model did not consider the work-system inputs/outputs, that is, inputs, information about risks and hazards that lead to MSDs and outputs, and information about the consequences of risk factor exposure. Axelsson's design [13] included work-systems and quality in a model of ergonomics. The model combined the concept of "fitness for use" developed by Juran [14] and the concepts in the book "Fitting the Task to the Man" developed by Grandjean [15]. His model based on Lemon's proposal considered only the work-system inputs, like interaction between the worker and the process, inside work space but did not include the outputs. Delgado-Bahena et al. proposed the Ergonomic Hazards Mapping System (EHMS). The model was developed using a rough layout in which the body parts exposed to hazards or risk factors were identified [16]. Nevertheless, their model only considers the work-system outputs and did not provide information on what leads to MSDs. It is important to consider that the models presented above contribute to understanding the ergonomic process problem, but they do not add information for detecting and preventing MSDs.

In the industrial context, a system comprises an interacting component collection that brings together common purposes; the system is limited by variables at any moment in time and is subject to a cause-effect mechanism [17]. The process mapping schematizes the system model using a pictorial relationship between variables. It is composed of legends, symbols, and scales explaining the interactions between system elements with the aim to identify the activities that add value [18]. It is divided into three parts: input-process-output, where the input connections or linkages among a selected part of a process (work system) transform the resources into another valued form (output). The process map represents the whole (end-to-end) work process [19]. Therefore, designs of ergonomic risk map based on the process map concept can contribute to identifying the risk of developing MSDs.

3. Case study

The workplace comprises three polish-screeners designed and built by company personnel, and they were used for polishing pieces of metal. The three machines polished around 50,000 pieces daily. The production time comprised three shifts of 8 h, with three operators per shift. The task was developed on a standing posture. Workers took a lunch time of 0.5 h, at the middle of the work period. Ergonomic risk factors like manual material handling, repetitive movements, awkward postures, and force exerted were to be identified as a part of task performance as is observed in **Table 2**.

	Task description	Repetition by shifts
	Barrel filling with: • Metal parts. • Corn cob powder.	44 times
	Sieve the corn cob powder from the metal parts. • Metal parts. • Fill a metallic bucket with metal polish using a manual metallic collector. • Fill the cardboard container with the polished metal.	2295 times
	Move the filled cardboard container to the inspection area.	310 times

Table 2.
Work method.

4. Ergonomic risk map design

To design the mapping, an analogy between the process map elements and ergonomic risks was developed. The relationship map regards the input/output connections or linkages among selected work tasks, and workstations were defined. The result is presented in **Table 3**.

The notations used for classifying the body segment affectation and the risk level of developing MSDs were based on the concept used by the ergonomic standards ISO 11228-3 [20] where the color identification for each risk level was as follows:

- Green—there is no risk of developing musculoskeletal disorders; a change in working conditions is unnecessary.

- Yellow—there is a risk of developing musculoskeletal disorders; a change in working conditions is needed.

- Red—there is a high risk of developing musculoskeletal disorders; a change in working conditions is needed immediately.

Information developed during the work-system assessment that can contribute to identifying risks that cause MSDs was organized according to the connections or linkages between ergonomic risk map elements as follows:
Inputs: work place conditions and human factors

- Work place design

- Nonergonomic task content

- Individual characteristics

Process components	Ergonomic risk map
Input	Information about risks and hazards that lead to MSDs • Work place conditions • Human factors
Process	Information about how the risk exposure leads to MSDs • Ergonomic risk factors present in the work place • Force demands
Output	Information about the consequences of risk factor exposure • Simple risk assessment results • Work-related injuries and illnesses • Cost of nonergonomics

Table 3.
Analogy between the process map elements and the ergonomic risk map elements.

Processes: ergonomic risk factors that cause MSDs and force demands by shift required to perform the task

- Weight manipulated

- Body segments affected

- Color identification of the risk level

- Force demands by shift required to perform the task measured in Newtons by movement

- Number of repetitions of the exertion strength

Outputs: risk assessment results, work-related illnesses, and the cost of nonergonomics

- Pain points in body segments

- Resume of task assessments

- Work-related injuries and illnesses

- Cost of nonergonomics

4.1 Method of construction

4.1.1 Inputs

Step 1. A list was made with risks or hazards that had been identified in a workplace, using data from assessment checklists. It should include only the workstation elements that limit the overall movement of the body or increase force requirements, causing pain or discomfort.

Step 2. A list was made with nonergonomic task elements, like awkward postures, repetitive movements, force exertion, and insufficient time recovery, among others.

Step 3. A list was made with individual characteristics that workers should change to prevent MSD development.

4.1.2 Process

Step 4. Photographs were added to identify the manipulated weight in each task element.

Step 5. Workstation layout was added. It represented machinery used for developing tasks.

Step 6. Images of body segments affected with color identification of the risk level were added.

Step 7. A list was made with force demands that caused pain/discomfort and exceeded the permissible standard value. It included isometric strength, leg lifting strength, grip strength, push and pull (initial force/kept force), and dynamic back extension strength, among others, in Newtons. The analysts were free to choose the measurement method that they consider most appropriate to complete this section.

Step 8. The number of repetitive exertions developed by workers was included.

4.1.3 Outputs

Step 9. A drawing of a body segment that identifies a point of pain was added. It represented the pain symptoms suffered by workers.

Step 10. All the simple risk assessments developed to determine the acceptability of risk were provided in one table. Identification of results with a color according to each risk level was obtained. REBA, NIOSH equation, and OCRA among others were included.

Step 11. All the work-related injuries or illnesses suffered by workers were categorized according to frequency in a Pareto chart.

Step 12. The cost of nonergonomics was estimated. It comprised workers with work-related injuries or illnesses, the daily salary (it included allowance for temporary inability and replacement worker salary), an average of lost workdays by a worker, and the total lost workdays per year.

5. Results and discussion

5.1 Analysis of inputs: work place conditions and human factors

5.1.1 Work place conditions

The ergonomic risk map was implemented in three polish-screener machines used for polishing pieces of metal; only nine workers were assigned to develop this task. The machines were poorly designed and built by engineers from the company. The workstation design did not consider basic anthropometric requirements, and this situation caused insufficient space for legs, incorrect working height and inconvenient arm reach, producing awkward postures that cause pain and discomfort.

5.1.2 Nonergonomic task content

With respect to nonergonomic task content, the risks found were as follows: exerting excessive force, similar task repetitively, doing work in awkward postures, being in the same posture for a long period, coming into contact with vibration surfaces, and manual handling—pushing and pulling loads and lifting and carrying loads; these conditions caused microtraumas that affect the body's recovery system of the workers.

5.1.3 Human factors

Moreover, individual characteristics like poor work practices, poor fitness, poor health habits, and poor work readiness add a probability of developing MSDs. Thus, programs about healthy life and better practices of manufacturing should be implemented.

5.2 Analysis of process: ergonomic risk factors that cause MSDs and force demands per shift required to perform the task

5.2.1 Weight manipulated

The work method included three task elements with manual handling—lifting and carrying loads:

1. Barrel filling with metal parts: a filled cardboard with 30 kg of weight is lifted over the shoulder 44 times, exerting an excessive force of around 277 N in each lifting,

2. sieving the corn cob powder from the metal parts: a filled metallic bucket containing metal polish with 20 kg of weight is handled 2295 times, exerting an excessive force of 77.62 N in each grip strength, and

3. moving filled cardboard containers with 80 kg of weight to an inspection area 310 times. Leg lifting strength of 143.20 N, dynamic back extension strength of 245.15 N, and push and pull (initial force/kept force) of 291/236 N, respectively, were considered in this force demands.

The task exceeds the biomechanical work load capacity of workers; this means that the musculoskeletal system suffers from fatigue and wears down in joints and muscle injuries. The workers have developed dorsopathies.

5.2.2 Body segments affected and color identification of the risk level

- Upper limbs—Red—there is a high risk of developing musculoskeletal disorders; the repetitive movements need to be eliminated immediately.

- Shoulders—Red—there is a high risk of developing musculoskeletal disorders; the height of the barrel need to be reduced immediately.

- Trunk (back)—Red—there is a high risk of developing musculoskeletal disorders; the conditions of manual material handling need to be changed immediately.

5.2.3 Force demands by shift required to perform the task measured in Newtons by movement and a number of repetitions of the exertion strength

The method used for the classification and definition of human muscular strength was proposed by Mital and Kumar [21], which divides the strength criteria into two sections: characteristics of the effort that include static isometric muscle strengths and isokinetic muscle strengths and characteristics of the application that include static functional strengths and dynamic functional strengths. The results obtained are summarized in **Table 4**.

5.3 Analysis of outputs

5.3.1 Pain points in body segments

In order to determine the pain points in body segments a questionnaire about MSD symptoms was to apply to the 9 operators of the three polish-screener machines. In the questionnaire the workers had to mark the body segment where they felt pain or had any injury. The resume of their answers is shown in **Figure 2**. The results do not correspond with the official information provided by the safety and health department used for building the Pareto chart developed for determined work-related injuries and illnesses (see Section 5.3.3).

5.3.2 Identification of task assessments

The results from the simple risk assessments were summarized in a table. In all the cases, the resulting risk levels were unacceptable. It allowed identifying the main unsafe and unhealthy task components. See **Figure 3**.

5.3.3 Work-related injuries and illnesses

The method employed to represent the work-related illnesses was the Pareto chart. It is a frequency distribution (or histogram). It was used for arranging injuries and illnesses by category. The Pareto method and rules of 70/30 (Pareto principle) allow identifying the main MSDs developed by workers in the work area. It can be used from the ergonomic intervention standpoint [22]. The information to build the Pareto chart was proportioned by the safety and health department. This official information indicates that all workers in the area (nine in total) have been suffering from almost two work-related injuries or illnesses (see **Figure 4**). It confirms the analysis developed in Section 5.2.1. However, it is contradictory with respect to workers' complaints. They identified the shoulder pain as the main

Classification	Measurement by movement (N)	No repetitions
Isometric shoulder strength	277.00	44
Leg lifting strength	143.20	310
Grip strength	77.62	2295
Push and pull (initial force/kept force)	291/236	310
Dynamic back extension strength	245.15	310

Table 4.
Force demands by shift required to perform the task.

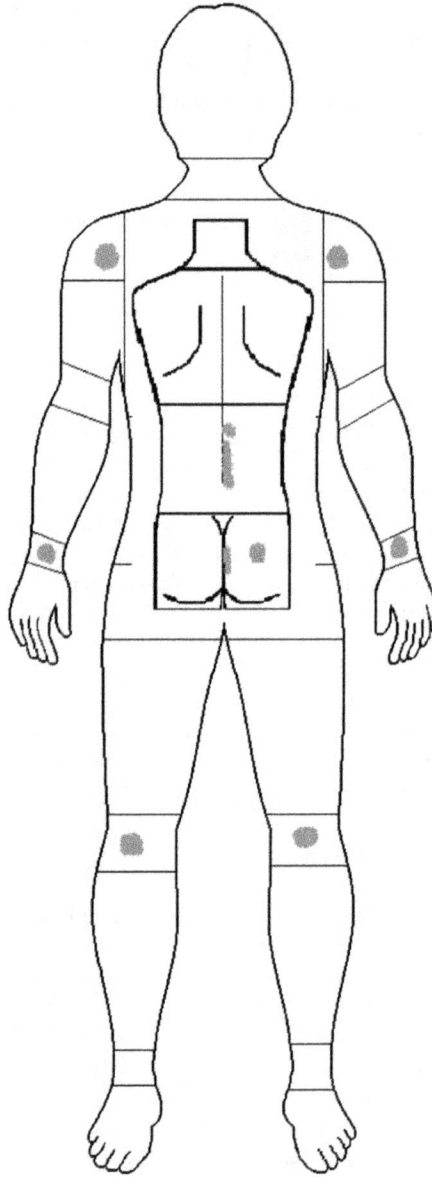

Figure 2.
Pain points in body segments selected by the workers through a questionnaire.

OCRA		X	
NIOSH			X
SNOOK and CIRIELLO			X
REBA			X
ADDITIONAL FACTORS			X
TIME RECOVERY			X

Figure 3.
Identification of task assessments.

Work-related injuries and illness in one year

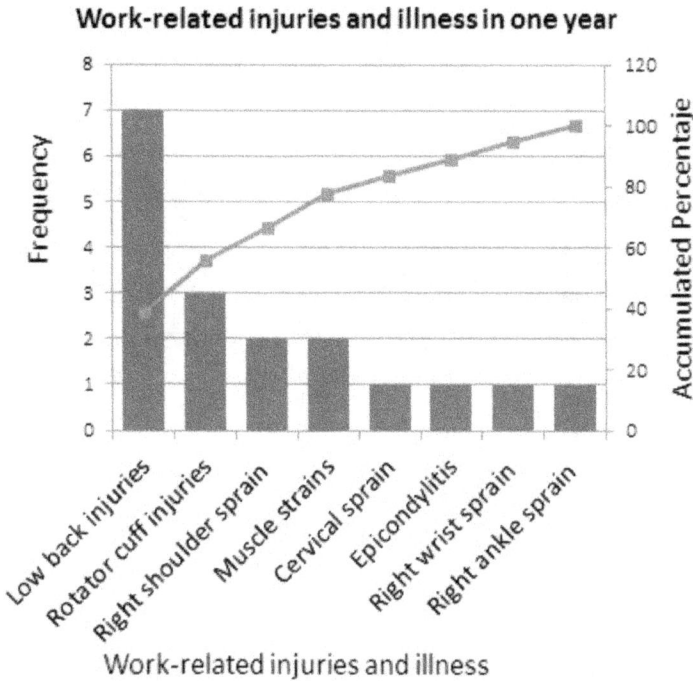

Figure 4.
Pareto chart about work-related injuries and illnesses.

symptom of MSDs. Thus, new studies to implement strategies to balance the differences of opinion are necessary.

5.3.4 Cost of nonergonomics

Workers with work-related injuries or illnesses: 18.
Daily salary: $34.63 USD (includes allowance for temporary inability).
Average of lost workdays by a worker: 35.
Total lost workdays per year: 630.
Total cost of nonergonomics: $392,704 USD ($7,461,380 MXP).
The resulting cost supports the suggestion to change the working method to eliminate repetitive movements, reduce the barrel height, and improve conditions about manual material handling.

5.4 Ergonomic risk map

All the information presented in previous sections was organized in a single spreadsheet. The ergonomic risk map shown in **Figure 5** summarizes result series derived from an exhaustive work place evaluation. The map added evidence necessary to determine that musculoskeletal disorders were caused by the workplace and incorrectly designed tasks. The resulting ergonomic risk map allowed to determine the causes of MSDs developed in activities in a three polish-screener, establishing the barrel height as a main cause of risk. The excessive height forces the material handling above the shoulders. This increases force demands required to perform the task. On the other hand, the work method must be changed in order to reduce repetitive movements. The map improves the employers'

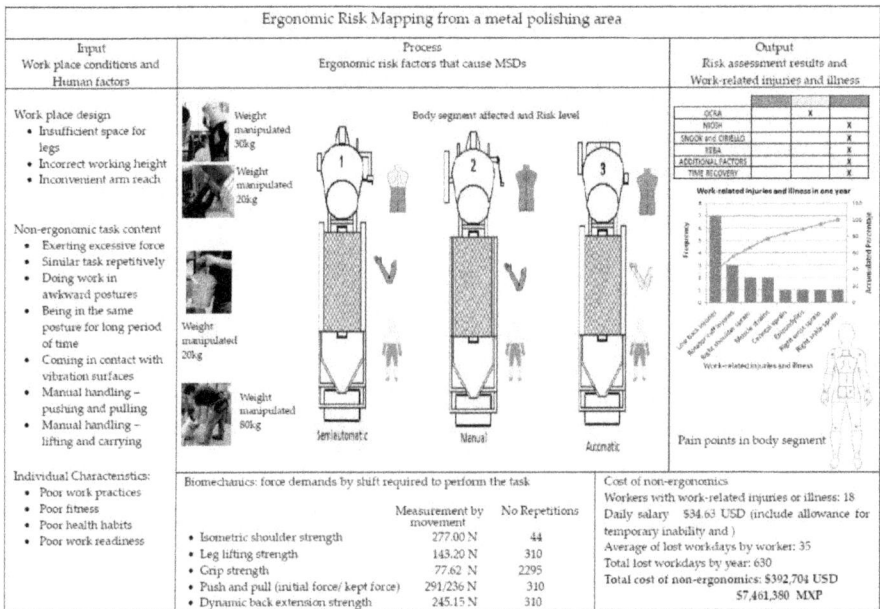

Figure 5.
Ergonomic risk map from three polish-screener machines.

understanding about the origin of ergonomic problems present in the polishing area and supports the decision-making about improvement projects focused on risk elimination.

6. Conclusions

The assessment and diagnosis method used for building an ergonomic risk map was developed and implemented with the objective of identifying the relationship, between the workplace design and the nonergonomic content task. The standardized method allows obtaining relevant diagnosis about hazards and ergonomic risks factors present in the work system that leads to musculoskeletal disorders. The study shows that the ergonomic risk map (a) improves the understanding of the workers and employers about the origin of ergonomic problems present in working areas, (b) identifies the main unsafe and unhealthy areas and work-system components, (c) supports the decision-making about improvement projects focused on risk elimination. However, the complaints and employers´ opinion in many cases were contradictory with respect to official information. Thus, new studies to implement strategies to balance the differences of opinion are necessary.

Acknowledgements

The authors are thankful to the company and its workers for their disposition, the Chemistry and Engineering College for its support, and industrial engineering students for their enthusiastic participation.

Author details

Martha Roselia Contreras-Valenzuela[1*], Alejandro David Guzmán-Clemente[1] and Francisco Cuenca-Jiménez[2]

1 Chemistry Sciences and Engineering College, Autonomous University of Morelos State, Cuernavaca, Morelos, Mexico

2 Engineering College, National Autonomous University of Mexico, Ciudad de México, Mexico

*Address all correspondence to: marthacv@uaem.mx

IntechOpen

References

[1] Mital A, Kumar S. Chapter 7. Human muscle strength definitions, measurement, and usage: Part I-guidelines for the practitioner. In: Ergonomic Guidelines and Problem Solving. In: Mital A, Kulbom A, Kumar S, editors. Elsevier Ergonomics Book Series Editors. Volume 1. UK, Kindlington: Oxford; 2000

[2] Budynas RG, Nisbett JK. Diseño en Ingeniería Mecánica de Shigley. Octava Edición ed. Mc Graw Hill. México: Mc Graw Hill Interamericana; 2008

[3] Arenas-Ortiz L, Cantú-Gómez O. Factores de Riesgo de trastornos músculo-esqueléticos crónicos laborales. Medicina Interna de México. 2013;29(4):370-379. Available from: http://www.imbiomed.com.mx/1/1/articulos.php?method=showDetail &id_articulo=94646&id_seccion=1479&id_ejemplar=9249&id_revista=47 [Accessed: 14-02-2018]

[4] Occupational Safety & Health Administration. Safety and Health Topics. Ergonomics [Internet]. USA. 2018. Available from: https://www.osha.gov/SLTC/ergonomics/ [Accessed: 25-01-2018]

[5] Cohen A, Gjessing C, Fine L, Bernard B, McGlothlin J. Element of Ergonomic Programs. A primer based on workplace evaluations of musculoskeletal disorders. DHHS (NIOSH) Publication No. 97-117. 1997. Available from: http://www.cdc.gov/niosh/docs/97-117/ [Accessed: 21-02-2018]

[6] Instituto Mexicano del Seguro Social (IMSS). Memoria Estadística [Internet]. Capítulo VII Salud en el Trabajo. 2017. Available at http://www.imss.gob.mx/conoce-al-imss/memoria-estadistica-2017 [Accessed: 01-06-2018]

[7] Secretaría del Trabajo y Previsión Social (STPS). Estadísticas del Sector. Riesgos de trabajo terminados registrados en el IMSS [Internet]. Available from: http://www.stps.gob.mx/gobmx/estadisticas/ [Accessed: 01-06-2018]

[8] Noriega M, Franco J, Garduño M, León L, Martínez S, Cruz A. Situación en México. Informe Continental sobre la Situación del Derecho a la Salud en el trabajo. Asociación Latinoamericana de Medicina Social Red de Salud y Trabajo. 2008. p. 174. Available from: http://www.alames.org/index.php/documentos/libros/medicina-social/informes/62-informe-continental-sobre-la-situacion-del-derecho-a-la-salud-en-el-trabajo [Accessed: 18-01-2018]

[9] Salinas-Tovar J, López-Rojas P, Soto-Navarro M, Caudillo- Araujo D, Sánchez-Román F, Borja-Aburto V. El subregistro potencial de accidentes de trabajo en el Instituto Mexicano del Seguro Social. Salud Pública de México. 2004;46(3):204-209. Available from: http://www.scielo.org.mx/scielo.php?script=sci_arttext&pid=S0036-36342004000300009 [Accessed: 18-01-2018]

[10] Secretaría del Trabajo y Previsión Social [Internet]. Los Factores de Riesgo Ergonómico. Boletín electrónico Trabajo Seguro. Año 11, No. 65 de octubre 2015. Available from: http://trabajoseguro.stps.gob.mx/trabajoseguro/boletines%20anteriores/2015/bol065/vinculos/2005-0795.htm [Accessed: 20-02-2018]

[11] Secretaría del Trabajo y Previsión Social–STPS. Reglamento Federal de Seguridad y Salud en el Trabajo [Internet]. 2014. Available from: http://asinom.stps.gob.mx:8145/upload/RFSHMAT.pdf [Accessed: 21-02-2018]

[12] Lemon TB. The organization of industrial ergonomics—A human machine model. Applied

Ergonomics;**11**:223-226. DOI:
10.1016/0003-6870(80)90232-X

[13] Axelsson J. Quality and ergonomics,
towards successful integration.
Doctoral dissertations in quality and
human-systems engineering. Sweden:
Linköping University; 2000

[14] Juran JM. Quality Control Handbook.
New York: McGraw-Hill; 1951

[15] Grandjean E. Fitting the Task to
the Man: A Textbook of Occupational
Ergonomics. First ed. London: Taylor
and Francis; 1988

[16] Delgado-Bahena M, Barrios-Perez
R, Contreras-Valenzuela M, Lopez-
Sesenes R. Ergonomic hazards mapping
system (EHMS) for musculoskeletal
disorders detection. In: Goossens
R, editor. Advances in Social &
Occupational Ergonomics. Advances in
Intelligent Systems and Computing. Vol.
487. Cham: Springer; 2017. pp. 377-386.
DOI: 10.1007/978-3-319-41688-5_35

[17] Smart NJ. Lean Biomanufacturing,
Creating Value through Innovative
Bioprocessing Approaches. First ed.
USA: Woodhead Publishing; 2013

[18] Bulutlar F, Kamasak R. Complex
adaptative leadership for performance:
A theoretical framework. In:
Proceedings: Springer Proceedings
in Complexity Book Series (SPCOM)
Chaos, Complexity and Leadership; 17
September 2013; 2012. pp 59-66. DOI:
10.1007/978-94-007-7362-2_9

[19] Damelio R. The Basics of Process
Mapping. Second ed. New York: CRC
Press Taylor and Francis Group; 2011.
ISBN: 139781439891278

[20] International Organization for
Standardization. International Standard
11228-3:2003(E), Ergonomics, Manual
Handling, Part 3. Handling of Low
Loads at High Frequency. 1st ed.
Switzerland: 2007

[21] Mital A, Sh K. Human muscle
strength definitions measurement
and usage: Part 1. Guidelines for the
practitioner. In: Ergonomic Guidelines
and Problem Solving Elsevier
Ergonomic Book Series. First ed. Vol. 1.
2000. pp. 103-122

[22] Miranda-Sánchez J, Contreras-
Valenzuela M. Development of the QOC
matrix—The worker's voice (Part 2).
In: Procedia Manufacturing Volume
3 Issue C. In Proceedings of the 6th
International Conference Applied
Human Factors and Ergonomics AHFE;
26-30 July 2015. pp. 4748-4755. DOI:
10.1016/j.promfg.2015.07.572

How Poor Workstation Design Causes Musculoskeletal Disorders: Research from QOC Matrix the Workers' Voice

Roy López Sesenes, Martha Roselia Contreras-Valenzuela,
Alber Eduardo Duque-Álvarez,
Alejandro David Guzmán-Clemente,
Viridiana Aydeé León-Hernández and
Francisco Cuenca-Jiménez

Abstract

An ergonomic intervention method based on QOC Matrix the workers' voice was implemented in a study case. The diagnosis and analysis developed are used in improvement proposals for workstation redesign. The workers' voice resulting from reports of the employee' complaints and symptomatology was the base for a standardized method that comprises: (a) QOC questionnaire application, (b) risk factor categorization, (c) determination of unsafe and unhealthy ergonomic metrics, (d) figuring out the task content impact in the workers' body, and (e) work system diagnosis. Since workers' voice, the risk identification made included: (1) the task content linked to work method: repetitiveness associated with the sensor activation using the fingers and the repetitive movements include twist and the stretch of wrist, (2) workplace design regarding container height and injuries caused in wrists and elbows due to hits, (3) task developed regarding risk time exposition and workers position, and (4) workplace design regards to housing collector distance from filling area linked to workers position adopted for reach bags. Improvements included redesign of the workstation with a system of 90° exit discharge curve, one elevation system, and a photoelectric sensor in filling nozzle for automatic filling. As an improvement result, the activity called bags provision was eliminated from the task.

Keywords: ergonomics, musculoskeletal disorders, ergonomic intervention, assessment, risk factors

1. Introduction

Physical and ergonomic risks cause musculoskeletal disorders (MSDs). Physical risks are external loads associated with long periods of exposure during tasks performed. The external loads are caused by awkward postures, manual material handling, repetitive motion, and force exerted. All of them are known as ergonomic risk factors (ERFs), which impact on health and well-being of workers [1, 2]. Ergonomics comprises a set of techniques directed to adequacy of the work to the people, optimizing human well-being and performing the overall system [3, 4]. Elements of work system are: workplace, tasks performed, tools manipulation, products and materials manipulation, work organization, and work environment [5, 6]. During the interaction of a person with the work system, unsafe and unhealthy elements must be changed or redesigned. The Mexican Ministry of Labor and Social Safety (STPS) defines that if one of this interaction is incorrectly designed, the work task requirements will become ERFs that can lead to musculoskeletal disorders and occupational illness [7].

In Mexico, the real number of musculoskeletal disorders (MSDs) developed by workers is unknown due to three main causes: (1) workers are afraid of being dismissed by employers if they report symptoms of illness [8], (2) employers have historically evaded the law and they have not usually implemented safety and health standards in workplaces [9], and (3) authorities have improperly followed up safety inspections. Therefore, the negligence triggered apathy to assure abatement of risk conditions and has caused omissions, contributing to under-reporting risk conditions and work accidents [10]. Despite under-reporting risk factors, the concern of Mexican authority is the upward trend of developing MSDs (within the industrial and service sectors), as established in the First Forum on Safety and Health at Work, carried out in Mexico City in August 2015, where the ergonomic risk factors are identified as a main problem due to their impact on workers' health and their economic costs [11]. The increase in cases (73% on average) in 8 years (2009–2017), informed by the Mexican Institute of Social Safety (IMSS) [12, 13], reported a cumulative total of 20,523 cases, identifying dorsopathies as the most prevalent work disease with 6752 cases (32.9%) followed by enthesopathies with 3490 cases (17.01%) and carpal tunnel syndrome with 3280 cases (15.9%) (**Figure 1**).

To abate this health problem, the government has issued a mandatory rule called Federal Rule for Safety and Health at Work (Reglamento Federal de Seguridad y Salud en el Trabajo) [14]. It includes employer obligations to find, to report, and to reduce ergonomic risks presented inside facilities. Thus, the question is: how

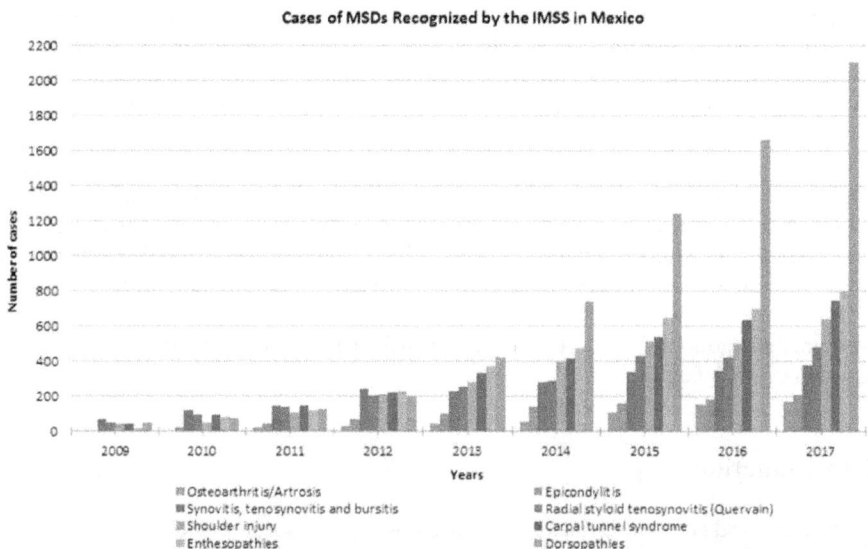

Figure 1.
Cases of MSDs reported by the IMSS during years 2009–2017 are organized according to the nature of injury.

employers can follow the law taking in to count that (a) ergonomic aspects are ignored for a long time, (b) ergonomic risks are seldom identified, and (c) an ergonomic intervention is not commonly carried out.

Based on the latter, it is important to define that an ergonomic intervention includes a diagnosis and analysis about the work system, which results in making improvement proposals [15]. If a proposal is carried out (elimination of ergonomic risk factors), a reduction of reports from employees' complaints must be observed.

In this chapter, an ergonomic intervention method based on QOC Matrix the workers' voice is carried out in a study case, the diagnosis and analysis developed were used to propose a workstation redesign as improvement proposals. Reports of the employees' complaints and symptomatology suffered represent the *workers' voice*. Improvement proposal should be standardized, to warranty workers' complaint reduction. Methods include: (a) QOC questionnaire application, (b) risk factor categorization, (c) determination of unsafe and unhealthy ergonomic metrics, (d) figuring out the task content impact in the workers' body, and (e) work system diagnosis.

2. Methods and tools

2.1 QOC Matrix the workers' voice ($_{QOC}$MWV)

QOC Matrix-the workers' voice ($_{QOC}$MWV) [16, 17] is an interactive ©Microsoft Excel spreadsheet. It uses decision support system (DSS) [18] that helps people to apply ergonomic parameters to identify and categorize the risk factors and fix them through ergonomic intervention.

It involves a *questionnaire* that encloses in each question *criteria* from: ergonomic ISO standards, Mexican safety and health standards, OSHA and NIOSH recommendations, among others used as evaluation parameters. During an ergonomic risk assessment, workers have to choose the *option* that answer questions according to their perception about workstation and tasks developed; the results got are called *workers' voice*.

The questionnaire was organized in to five sections: (1) work area with two subdivisions: (a) workplace design and (b) task content, (2) manual material handling, (3) work organization, (4) work environment, and (5) psychosocial aspects. Metrics for intervention and specific risk factors are obtained because of its implementation. Metrics are proportions (%) that define the level of risk. Specific risk factors are dimensional relations worker-workstation, repetitiveness, load manipulated, and exposition time. The results are represented in Pareto charts.

2.2 Pareto charts

Pareto chart is a frequency distribution (or histogram). It was used for arranging risk factors by category. Pareto method and rules of 70/30 (Pareto principle) [19] can identify crucial areas from the intervention standpoint. When the Pareto principle is determined, the common effect of workers' answers that a relative few of the contributors (risk factors)—the vital few—accounts for the bulk of the effect (MSDs). The vital few identification is easier when the tabular data are presented in graphic form that encloses the next main elements [20]:

1. Risk factors to the total effect, ranked by the magnitude of their contribution

2. Magnitude of each risk factor is expressed as a percentage of total

3. Sum of magnitude of all contributors is expressed as a total percentage.

3. Case study

The $_{QOC}$MWV survey was implemented in three automatic high-speed lines designed for filling dialysis bags with a liquid mixture and produces 110,000 bags daily. The production time comprised three shifts of 8 h, with 16 operators in each line by shift. Activities were developed on standing posture. Workers took a lunch time of 0.5 h, in the middle of the work period. Ergonomic risk factors like manual material handling, repetitive movements, awkward postures, and force exerted were identified as a part of task performance. In **Table 1**, the work method developed by a worker is presented.

Because of exceeding permissible exposure limits by operators, the company has received a preaction for probable occupational disease ST-9 (official document) issued by the IMSS, to the medical treatment for work-related injuries and diseases. In a preanalysis, the following percentage of cases suffered by workers was found: 30% epicondylitis, 20% hand tendinitis, and 10% shoulder injury.

Activity	Left hand	Right hand
Bags provision (92 × shift)	1. Reach housing collector to grasp 30–50 bags (the amount of grasped bags depends on worker skills) 2. Move the bags to the container 3. Arrange the bags and put in right position 4. Release the bags in container	1. Wait for bags 2. Hold the bags 3. Hold the bags 4. Release the bags
Fill bag (4584 bags per person)	1. Take bag no. 1 from container 2. Position the bag pipe under filling spout 3. Hold bag with fingers 4. Hold bag with fingers until filling starts 5. Wait 6. Hold filled bag with fingers 7. Position filled bag with fingers 8. Take bag no. 2 from container	1. Put up in filling spout 2. Activate filling with the little finger 3. Take balloon port from container 4. Soak balloon port in glue 5. Position balloon port 6. Put balloon port in filled bag 7. Release filled bag

Table 1.
Work method used to fill dialysis bag.

4. Method for ergonomic intervention

The method used for implementing the ergonomic intervention was applied as follows:

Step 1: the workers' voice was collected through applying QOC questionnaires.
Step 2: the results of workers' voice were the base to categorize ergonomic risk factors, through a Pareto chart in three cases of intervention:

1. effects caused in workplace by unsafe and unhealthy elements,

2. effects caused in work task by unsafe and unhealthy elements,

3. task content impacts in the workers' body.

Step 3: once the risk factors were identified, an ergonomic work system diagnosis was carried out.

Step 4: project improvements were determined to abate risk factors identified.

5. Results and discussions

5.1 Work system diagnosis

Questionnaire $_{QOC}$MWV was applied to 48 operators and three supervisors from each shift. (In **Figure 2**, an example of part of assessment is shown.) Workers tested the work system, and the task was chosen from options. Options were represented

No.	QUESTIONS	1	2	3	4	5
	WORKERS' VOICE N= UNCONFORTABLE / N= NO NT= NOT AT ALL CONFORTABLE / NT= NOT AT ALL = NO DEL TODO S= CONFORTABLE / S= YES = SI					
	1. WORK AREA					
	1.1 WORK PLACE DESIGN					
1	Does the work area suitable to the operator according to his/her physical conditions?	N	N	N	NT	N
2	Do the head and hips movements easy and safety?	NT	N	NT	NT	S
3	Do the movements of the feet in comfortable position?	NT	NT	N	NT	S
4	There are some mechanisms which allowed to manipulate higher loads (more than 50kg like hoist/ platforms, etc)?	N	N	N	N	N
	1.2 TASK CONTENT					
5	Does the work task not have repetitive movements which can cause fatigue in arms, shoulders, forearm and wrists?	N	N	N	N	N
6	Does manual manipulation not have repetitive movements and does no require a major force to lift a load in which involves distance and time that causes stress on the trunk and lower limbs?	N	N	N	N	N
7	Do the machinery and/or process not determine the rhythm of work?	S	S	S	S	S
8	Do the handles or slings help to manipulate the materials in easy way and they are well located?	N	NT	NT	N	S
	2. MATERIALS					
9	Is there a place assigned for each tool, machinery and row material?	S	S	S	S	S
10	Is the process free of machinery or tools vibrations?	N	N	N	N	N
11	Does product manipulated at room temperature?	N	N	N	N	N
	3. WORK ORGANIZATION					
12	Were you trained to perform the task?	S	S	S	S	S
13	Is there a procedure in which specifies the ergonomic requirements of the workstation and tasks?	N	N	N	N	N
14	Is there a work method that establishes unsafe and unhealthy activities?	N	N	N	N	N
15	Do you periodically receive medical review inside facility?	S	S	S	S	S
16	Do you practice labor gymnastics during the task?	N	N	N	N	N
17	Does the task not require activities such as planning, inspecting or correcting?	S	S	S	S	S
18	Do you finish you work on time and you do not require over time?	S	S	S	S	S
19	Define you task as follows: Y= light, NT=moderate, N=heavy	N	N	N	N	NT
	4. WORK ENVIRONMENT					
20	The lighting can enhance task performance allows observing the details of the product/material and does not generate shadows?	NT	NT	N	N	S
21	Does the work area clean and in optimal conditions to perform the demanded task?	S	S	NT	S	S
22	Does the noise allow speaking without shouting?	N	N	N	N	N
24	Do you consider the temperature of work place is comfortable to work?	N	NT	NT	NT	Y
	5. PSYCOSOCIAL ASPECTS					
25	Do you not do high speed activities or activities that need a lot concentration?	N	N	N	N	N
26	Do you feel motivated at work and without pressure and stress?	S	S	NT	N	S

Figure 2.
Example of a questionnaire applied using the QOC matrix—the workers' voice.

Symbol	Description	Color	Risk associated
S = Yes	Comfortable	Green	No risk
NT = Not at all	Not at all comfortable	Yellow	Risk
N = No	Uncomfortable	Red	High risk

Table 2.
Options chosen during the evaluation using $_{QOC}$MWV.

by letters that symbolized a level of comfort, for example, "S" for comfortable. Each option was associated with a color to show the risk [21], as shown in **Table 2**.

In Mexico, the workforce is people who have basic studies in the best case; therefore, workers' training is difficult in ergonomics issues. Therefore, the survey made to the workers focuses in their filings, complaints, and motivations [16]. The matrix results were organized through three Pareto chart.

5.2 Categorization of ergonomic risk factors

5.2.1 Unsafe elements of work system components

Figure 3 shows the work system elements evaluated. According to Pareto principle, the cumulated frequency symbolizes "the vital few" (see Section 2.2). Therefore, this percentage was considered as the workers' voice index. Unfortunately, the Pareto principle was not presented in the first chart (rule of 70/30) as is observed in **Figure 3**, due to which there were small differences between opinions about unsafe and unhealthy work system elements. Workplace and task content received 18 complaints, each one representing only 37% of cumulate frequency, and materials handling and psychosocial factors received 17 complaints, each one representing only 35.06% of cumulate frequency, the 70% was to reach until the fourth bar and not in the first three bars, as established by the Pareto rule. Hence, there was no main work system element identified as workers' voice to be improved during the intervention.

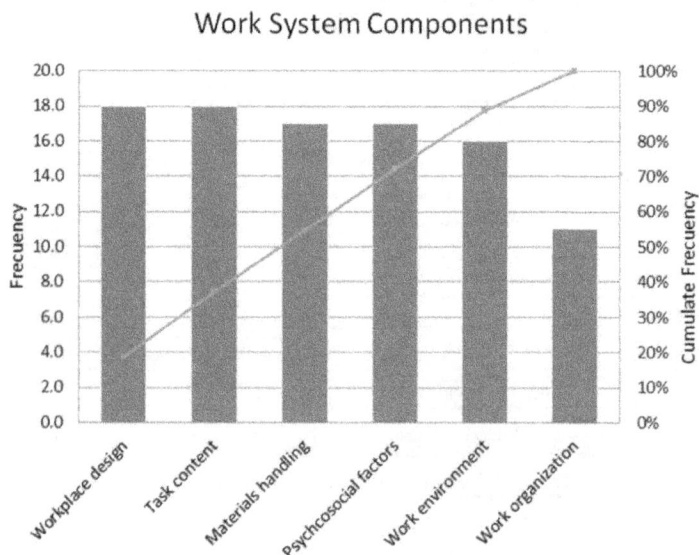

Figure 3.
Pareto chart resulted from work system components evaluation.

The unusual behavior got in the Pareto chart was explained by the workers' complaints in this manner; *workplace design:* the workers suffered continuous little hits in wrists and elbows, caused by the container height and the housing collector distance from filling area, arm overstretching in the moment of taking set bags, and awkward position during the filling bag process. *Task content and materials handling:* as the speed of line was too fast, and they have to handle huge materials quickly and exhaustively. Aspects were confirmed with the results got in the second Pareto chart.

5.2.2 Unsafe and unhealthy ergonomic metrics

In the second Pareto chart, the ergonomic metrics about the task were evaluated, see **Figure 4**. The chart bars symbolize the task metrics, which was assessed by the QOCMWV by comparing the process parameters vs. international standards. In this chart, the Pareto principle was more clearly presented (rule of 70/30). Unfavorable environment received 23 complaints, repetitiveness received 20 complaints, and body position received 19, thus representing only 64% of cumulate frequency, close to 70%. Hence, unfavorable environment, repetitiveness, and body position were identified as workers voice to be improved during the intervention.

The chart results due to the unfavorable environment of the task were tied with the workplace design, and then at least 41 opinions from the 48 workers had complaints about work place design; in the same way, task content was linked with repetitiveness; then, at least 40 from the 48 workers had complaints about task content. Thus, *workplace design* and *task content* were identified as *workers' voice*.

5.2.3 How task content impacts workers´ body

In the third Pareto chart, the task content impact in the workers' body was assessed. The chart bars that represent the human body parts were exposed to injury due to ergonomic hazards and unsafe conditions. Once again, the Pareto principle was not presented in the third chart (rule of 70/30) as observed in **Figure 5**. However, the upper limbs (as a whole) were identified as affected by the repetitive works developed.

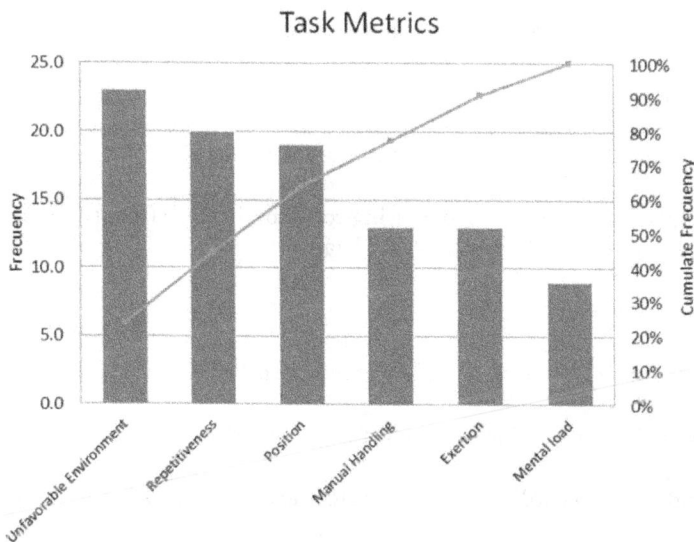

Figure 4.
Pareto chart resulted from task metrics identified as risk.

Body parts with probable MSDs development

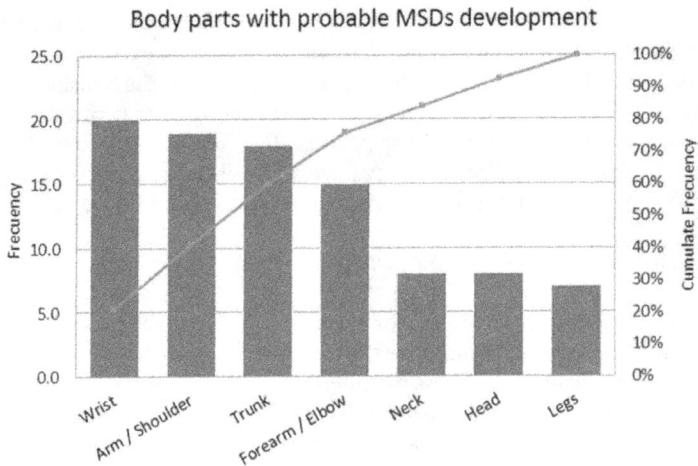

Figure 5.
Pareto chart representation of body parts identified that will probably be injured.

5.3 Diagnosis to determine the incompliances regarding ergonomic rules

The results of the diagnosis about incompliance of ergonomic rules inside the work system are mentioned below.

5.3.1 Identification of risks

1. The task content about work method:

   a. Repetitiveness associated with the sensor activation using the fingers

   b. The repetitive movements include twist and the stretch of wrist

2. Workplace design regards to container height:

   a. Injuries associated with wrists and elbows hits

3. Task content regards to task duration about workers' position

4. Workplace design regards to housing collector distance from filling area about workers' position adopted for reach bags.

5.3.2 Symptoms found

1. Wrist pain and swelling caused by repetitive little hits

2. Elbow pain and swelling caused by repetitive little hits

3. Shoulder pain regarding arm overstretching position adopted to reach bags

4. Back pain regarding task duration and workers' position adopted to reach bags.

5.4 Improving proposal work station redesign

5.4.1 Transport system of bags

In order to eliminate the 92 repeated overstretching positions taken by the workers during task performance (**Table 1**), redesign of the workstation was proposed (see **Figure 6**). Improving proposal included a transport system of a 90° exit discharge curve, which will position in the right way the bags are directed into the base container. Regarding poor design of container height and the distance between the collector and the worker, a slide elevator system was added, which included an optical sensor with two main functions. First one consists in detecting each bag to move the elevator system down when each bag is deposited in the container base, the second one refers to moving up the container base added to the elevator system when a determinate quantity of bags is counted, allowing the workers to reach without additional efforts to the bags. Additionally, a synchronization of the conveyor system was suggested, improving the productivity and decreasing the overwork driving to the human factor.

5.4.2 Photoelectric sensor implementation in filling nozzle

For reducing repetitiveness in the activation sensor (**Table 1**) during filling bag (right hand), a photoelectric sensor was implemented. It will automatically activate the filling nozzle. This implementation allowed eradicating the twist and stretch movements generated at wrist (see **Figure 7**).

5.4.3 Work method improvements

After ergonomic intervention, "bags provision" activity (**Table 1**) was eliminated, as well as the activation of filling with right-hand little finger. The work method resulting is shown in **Table 3**.

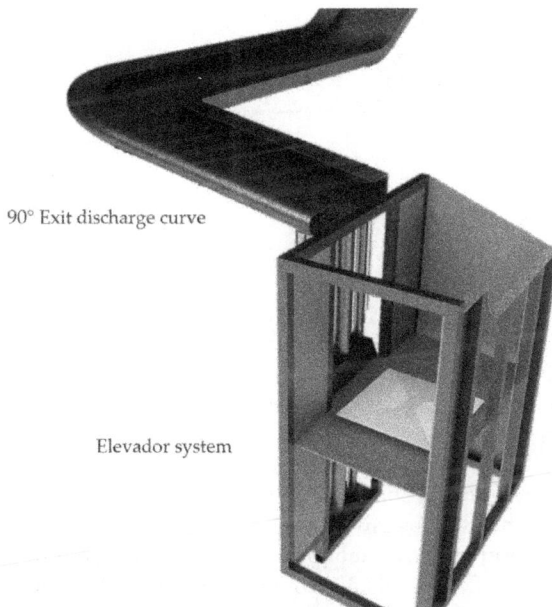

90° Exit discharge curve

Elevador system

Figure 6.
Workstation proposed redesign. It includes a system transport of 90° exit discharge curve and an elevation system.

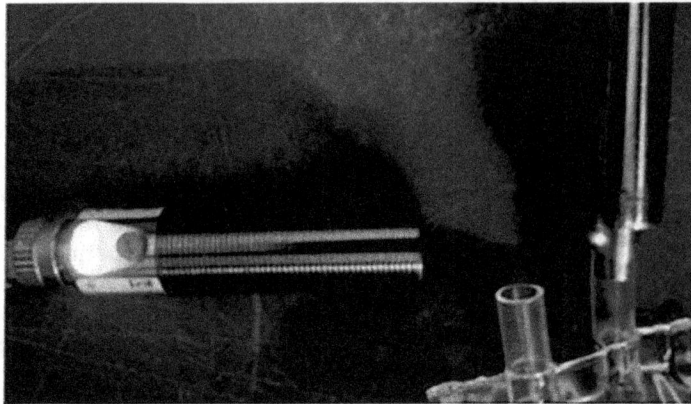

Figure 7.
Photoelectric sensor in filling nozzle for automatic filling.

Activity	Left hand	Right hand
Fill bag (5000 bags per person) 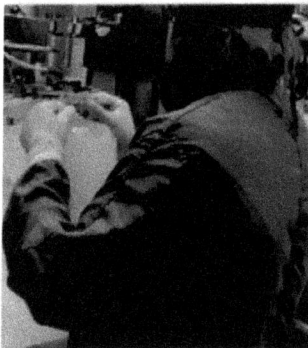	1. Take bag no. 1 from container 2. Position bag under filling spout 3. Hold bag with fingers 4. Hold bag with fingers until filling starts 5. Wait 6. Hold filled bag with fingers 7. Take bag no. 2 from container	8. Put up in filling spout 9. Take balloon port from container 10. Soak balloon port in glue 11. Position balloon port 12. Put balloon port in filled bag 13. Release filled bag

Table 3.
New work method for the task filling dialysis bag.

6. Conclusions

The assessment and diagnosis method based on $_{QOC}$MWV was developed and implemented, with the objective of improving the labor relationship, between workers and employers as well as their working conditions. The standardized method allows obtaining relevant diagnosis about hazards and ergonomic risks factors present in the work system, which leads to musculoskeletal disorders. The study shows that the $_{QOC}$MWV: (a) improves the worker-employer understanding about origin of ergonomic problems present in working areas, (b) identifies the main unsafe and unhealthy areas and work system components, (c) supports the decision-making about improvement projects focused on risk elimination, (d) the workers´ fear of being dismissed by employers if they report symptoms of illness was diminished because the survey was anonymous. However, the workers' voice (complains) and the employers´ opinion in many cases were contradictory. Thus, it is necessary for new studies to implement strategies to balance the differences in opinion.

Acknowledgements

We appreciate the enthusiastic participation of the employees who take part in the evaluation as well as the company contribution in the development of this study.

Author details

Roy López Sesenes[1], Martha Roselia Contreras-Valenzuela[1*], Alber Eduardo Duque-Álvarez[1], Alejandro David Guzmán-Clemente[1], Viridiana Aydeé León-Hernández[1] and Francisco Cuenca-Jiménez[2]

1 Chemistry Sciences and Engineering College, Autonomous University of Morelos State, Cuernavaca, Morelos, Mexico

2 Engineering College, National Autonomous University of Mexico, Ciudad de México, Mexico

*Address all correspondence to: marthacv@uaem.mx

IntechOpen

References

[1] Parra M. Conceptos básicos en salud laboral. Textos de capacitación. In: Central Unilateral de Trabajadores de Chile. Santiago: Oficina Internacional del Trabajo; 2003. ISBN 92-2-314530-X

[2] Singleton WT. The Nature and Aims of Ergonomics, Encyclopedia of Occupational Health and Safety. Part IV Tools & Approaches. International Labor Organization [Internet]. 2011. Available from: http://www.iloencyclopaedia.org/part-iv-66769/ergonomics-52353/goals-principles-and-methods-91538/goals/the-nature-and-aims-of-ergonomics [Accessed: 25-01-2018]

[3] International Organization for Standardization. International Standard 6385:2004(E), Ergonomic Principles in the Design of Work Systems. 2nd ed. Switzerland: ISO; 2004

[4] Occupational Safety & Health Administration. Safety and Health Topics. Ergonomics [Internet]. 2018. Available from: https://www.osha.gov/SLTC/ergonomics/ [Accessed: 25-01-2018]

[5] Attwood D, Deeb J, Danz-Reece M. Ergonomic Solutions for the Process Industries. USA: Gulf Professional Publishing, Elsevier; 2004. p. 480. DOI: 10.1016/ B978-0-7506-7704-2.X5000-4

[6] Cohen A, Gjessing C, Fine L, Bernard B, McGlothlin J. Element of Ergonomic Programs. A Primer Based on Workplace Evaluations of Musculoskeletal Disorders. DHHS (NIOSH) Publication No. 97-117. 1997. Available from: http://www.cdc.gov/niosh/docs/97-117/ [Accessed: 21-02-2018]

[7] Secretaría del Trabajo y Previsión Social—STPS. Mexican Official Standard PROY-NOM-036-1-STPS-2017. Factores de riesgo ergonómico en el trabajo-Identificación, análisis, prevención y control. Parte 1- Manejo manual de cargas [Internet]. Available from: http://www.dof.gob.mx/nota_detalle.php?codigo=5510064&fecha=04/01/2018 [Accessed: 25-01-2018]

[8] Arenas-Ortiz L, Cantú-Gómez O. Factores de Riesgo de trastornos músculo-esqueléticos crónicos laborales. Medicina Interna de México. 2013;**29**(4):370-379. Available from: http://www.imbiomed.com.mx/1/1/articulos.php?method=showDetail&id_articulo=94646&id_seccion=1479&id_ejemplar=9249&id_revista=47 [Accessed: 14-02-2018]

[9] Noriega M, Franco J, Garduño M, León L, Martínez S, Cruz A. Situación en México. Informe Continental sobre la Situación del Derecho a la Salud en el trabajo. Asociación Latinoamericana de Medicina Social Red de Salud y Trabajo. 2008. p. 174. Available from: http://www.alames.org/index.php/documentos/libros/medicina-social/informes/62-informe-continental-sobre-la-situacion-del-derecho-a-la-salud-en-el-trabajo [Accessed: 18-01-2018]

[10] Salinas-Tovar J, López-Rojas P, Soto-Navarro M, Caudillo-Araujo D, Sánchez-Román F, Borja-Aburto V. El subregistro potencial de accidentes de trabajo en el Instituto Mexicano del Seguro Social. Salud Pública de México. 2004;**46**(3):204-209. Available from: http://www.scielo.org.mx/scielo.php?script=sci_arttext&pid=S0036-36342004000300009 [Accessed: 18-01-2018]

[11] Secretaría del Trabajo y Previsión Social. Los Factores de Riesgo Ergonómico. Boletín electrónico Trabajo Seguro [Internet]. Año 11, No. 65 de octubre 2015. Available from: http://trabajoseguro.stps.gob.mx/trabajoseguro/boletines%20

anteriores/2015/bol065/
vinculos/2005-0795.htm [Accessed:
20-02-2018]

[12] Instituto Mexicano del Seguro
Social (IMSS). Memoria Estadística
2017, Capítulo VII Salud en el Trabajo
[Internet]. Available at http://www.
imss.gob.mx/conoce-al-imss/memoria-
estadistica-2017 [Accessed: 01-06-2018]

[13] Secretaría del Trabajo y Previsión
Social (STPS). Estadísticas del Sector.
Riesgos de trabajo terminados registrados
en el IMSS [Internet]. Available from:
http://www.stps.gob.mx/gobmx/
estadisticas/ [Accessed: 01-06-2018]

[14] Secretaría del Trabajo y Previsión
Social—STPS. Reglamento Federal
de Seguridad y Salud en el Trabajo
[Internet]. 2014. Available from: http://
asinom.stps.gob.mx:8145/upload/
RFSHMAT.pdf [Accessed: 21-02-2018]

[15] Castillo-Martínez JA. Ergonomía,
fundamentos para el desarrollo de
soluciones ergonómicas. Colombia:
Universidad del Rosario; 2010. p. 215.
ISBN-10: 9587380932

[16] Lozano-Ramos E, Contreras-
Valenzuela M. Development of the QOC
Matrix—The worker's voice (Part 1).
Advances in social and organizational
factors. In: Proceedings of the 5th
International Conference Applied
Human Factors and Ergonomics AHFE;
19-23 July 2014. pp. 433-440

[17] Miranda-Sánchez J, Contreras-
Valenzuela M. Development of the QOC
matrix—The worker's voice (Part 2).
In: Procedia Manufacturing Volume
3 Issue C. In Proceedings of the 6th
International Conference Applied
Human Factors and Ergonomics AHFE;
26-30 July 2015. pp. 4748-4755. DOI:
10.1016/j.promfg.2015.07.572

[18] Power DJ. Decision Support
Systems: Concepts and Resources for
Managers. 1st ed. USA: Quorum Books:
Greenwood Publishing Group Inc.;
2002. p. 261. ISBN: 1-56720-497-X

[19] Juran JM, Godfrey AB. Juran's
Quality Handbook. 5th ed. USA:
McGraw Hill; 1999. p. 1700

[20] Montgomery Duglas C. Introduction
to Statistical Quality Control. 6th ed.
USA: John Wiley & Sons, Inc.; 2009.
p. 754

[21] International Organization for
Standardization. International Standard
11228-1:2003(E), Ergonomics, Manual
Handling, Part 1. Lifting and Carrying.
1st ed. Switzerland: ISO; 2003

Diagnosis and Treatment
of WRMSDs

Chapter 4

De Quervain's Tenosynovitis: Effective Diagnosis and Evidence-Based Treatment

Jenson Mak

Abstract

De Quervain's tenosynovitis (DQT) is a repetitive stress condition located at the first dorsal compartment of the wrist at the radial styloid. The extensor pollicis brevis (EPB) and abductor pollicis longus (APL) tendons and each tendon sheath are inflamed and this may result in thickening of the first dorsal extensor sheath. Workers who perform repetitive activities of the wrist and hand and those who routinely use their thumbs in grasping and pinching motions in a repetitive manner are most susceptible to DQT. Conservative treatments include activity modification, modalities, orthotics, and manual therapy. This chapter identifies, in an evidence base manner through the literature, the most effective diagnostic measures for DQT. It also examines the evidence base on (or lack thereof) the treatment or treatment combinations to reduce pain and improve functional outcomes for patients with DQT.

Keywords: De Quervain's tenosynovitis, diagnosis, treatment, workplace, evidence-based

1. Introduction

In 1893, Paul Jules Tillaux described a painful crepitus sign (Aïe crépitant de Tillaux)—tenosynovitis of the adductor and the short extensor of the thumb. In 1894, Fritz de Quervain, a Swiss surgeon, first described tenosynovitis on December 18, 1894, in Mrs. D., a 35-year-old woman who had severe pain in the extensor muscle region of the thumb, excluding tuberculosis.

"It is a condition affecting the tendon sheaths of the abductor pollicis longus, and the extensor pollicis brevis. It has definite symptoms and signs. The condition may affect other extensor tendons at the wrist" [1].

Patients with DQT have difficulty gripping objects and performing their daily activities. De Quervain's tendinopathy affects the abductor pollicis longus (APL) and extensor pollicis brevis (EPB) tendons in the first extensor compartment at the styloid process of the radius. It is characterized by pain or tenderness at the radial side of the wrist. Although de Quervain's tendinopathy is often attributed to overuse or repetitive movements of the wrist or thumb, the cause is generally unknown.

2. Epidemiology

De Quervain's tenosynovitis (DQT) is a common cause of wrist pain in adults and is the second most common entrapment tendinopathy in the hand following trigger finger. It usually occurs in middle-aged individuals and is around 3× more common in women (~80% of cases). It is most common among women between the ages of 30 and 50 years of age, including a small subset of women in the postpartum period [2]. These women tend to develop symptoms about 4–6 weeks after delivery. In a large analysis of a young active population of military personnel, women again had a significantly higher rate of de Quervain's tenosynovitis at 2.8 cases per 1000 person-years, compared to men at 0.6 per 1000 person-years (almost 5×). Age greater than 40 was also a significant risk factor, with this age category showing a rate of 2.0 per 1000 person-years compared to 0.6 per 1000 in personnel under 20 years. There was also a racial difference, with blacks affected at 1.3 per 1000 person-years compared to whites at 0.8, in this population [3].

With regard to work, Stahl found that in 189 patients surgically treated for DQT vs. 198 patients with wrist ganglia (WG) (controls), there was no significant difference between DQT vs. WG found after subgrouping professional activities (manual labor: 18 vs. 26%, respectively, p = 0.23). In addition, there was no asymmetric distribution of comorbidities, wrist trauma, forceful or repetitive manual work, or medication observed, and it was concluded that neither heavy manual labor nor trauma could be shown to be predisposing risk factors for DQT (**Figure 1**). Most cases of DQT, however, are associated with overuse, and, local trauma can also precipitate the condition [4].

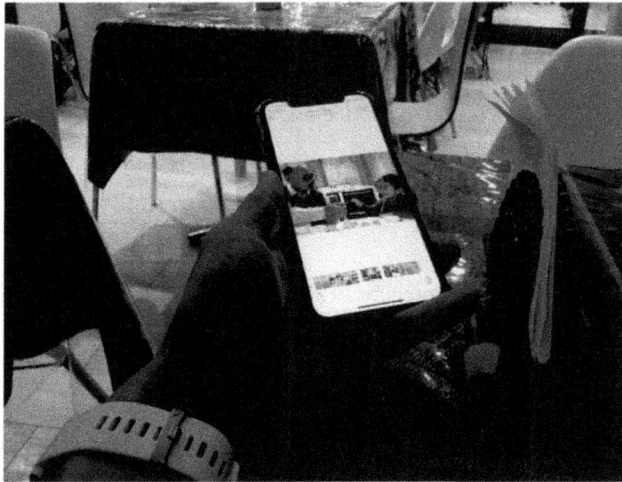

Figure 1.
De Quervain's tenosynovitis (DQT) is one of the most common work-related upper limb musculoskeletal disorders especially in the age of smartphones, tablets and laptop devices.

3. Pathophysiology

The etiology of de Quervain's tenosynovitis (DQT) is not well understood. In the past, it was frequently attributed to occupational or repetitive activities involving postures that maintain the thumb in extension and abduction. As an example, it has been thought that new mothers are at risk postpartum due to repetitive motion of hands required to lift and hold newborns. Hormonal causes and fluid retention are another plausible explanation. The evidence to support etiologic hypotheses is limited and is largely based on observational data. The histopathology does not demonstrate inflammation but rather myxoid degeneration (disorganized collagen and increased cellular matrix) in patients referred for surgery [5].

DQT affects both the abductor pollicis longus (APL) and the extensor pollicis brevis (EPB) at the point where they pass through a fibro-osseous tunnel (the first dorsal compartment) from the forearm into the hand. These tendons are responsible for bringing the thumb away from the hand as it lies flat in the plane of the palm (i.e., radial abduction). Similar to trigger finger (or stenosing flexor tenosynovitis), this disease involves a noninflammatory thickening of both the tendons and the tunnel (or sheath) through which they pass. The APL and EPB tendons are tightly secured against the radial styloid by the overlying extensor retinaculum which creates a fibro-osseous tunnel. Thickening of the retinaculum and tendons from acute or repetitive trauma restrains normal gliding within the sheath. This causes inflammation and further edematous thickening of the tendon exacerbating the local stenosing effect. Microscopically, there are inflammatory cells found within the tendon sheath.

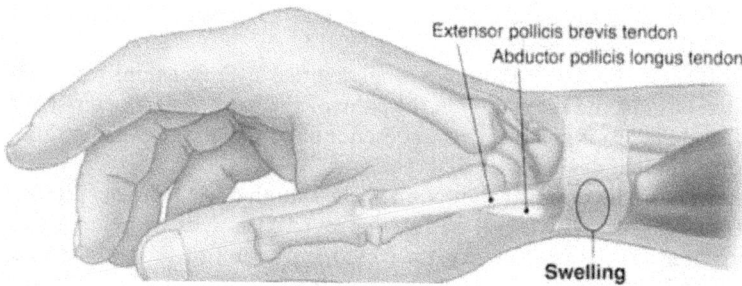

In ~10% of patients, there is an intertendinous septum between APL and EPB. The absence of a septum is associated with very high rates (almost 100%) of complete symptom resolution with conservative management. Presence of an intertendinous septum increases the likelihood that surgical management will be required.

Stahl et al. [6] reviewed in a meta-analysis of 80 articles of an association between DQT and (1) repetitive, (2) forceful, or (3) ergonomically stressful manual work suggesting an odds ratio of 2.89 (95% CI, 1.4–5.97; p = 0.004). The analysis, however, found no evidence to support the Bradford Hill criteria for a causal relationship between de Quervain's tenosynovitis and occupational risk factors.

4. Evidence-based review

While there have been several multidisciplinary treatment guidelines published [7], they are consensus-based rather than evidence-based. This review seeks to address this issue and identify any gaps in research for the investigation and treatment of DQT.

Systematic search of MEDLINE, CINAHL and EMBASE for articles published from September 2014 to August 2018, and the Cochrane Database of Systematic Reviews (most recent issue searched—Issue 2, 2018). Randomized controlled trials, meta-analyses, and reviews of all aspects of diagnoses and treatment for DQT among participants were limited to those aged 18 years.

All studies were reviewed independently by the author, who recorded individual study results, and an assessment of study quality and treatment conclusions was made according to evidence-based protocols.

Out of a total of 72 articles from PUBMED for DQT diagnosis, we found 10 articles satisfying the research criteria. There were no suitable Cochrane review articles.

Out of a total of 95 articles from PUBMED for DQT treatment, we found 20 articles satisfying the criteria. There were no suitable Cochrane review articles.

5. Evidence-based DQT diagnosis

5.1 Clinical examination diagnosis

The Finkelstein test (**Figure 2**) is named after Harry Finkelstein (1865–1939), an American surgeon who first described it in 1930. It is a clinical test used to assess the presence of DQT in people with wrist pain. It is performed by grasping the patients thumb and deviating the hand in the ulnar direction. If a sharp pain occurs along the distal radius, this is considered to make DQT likely.

Eichhoff's test (**Figure 3**) is often wrongly named as Finkelstein's test. Eichhoff's test consists of grasping the thumb in the palm of the hand while the wrist is ulnar deviated, and the test is positive in the presence of pain over the radial styloid process during lunar deviation of the wrist.

The wrist hyperflexion and abduction of the thumb (WHAT) test (**Figure 4**) revealed greater sensitivity (0.99) and an improved specificity (0.29) together with a slightly better positive predictive value (0.95) and an improved negative predictive value (0.67) compared with Eichhoff's test in one study [8]. Moreover, the study showed that the wrist hyperflexion and abduction of the thumb test was very valuable in diagnosing dynamic instability after successful decompression of the first extensor compartment.

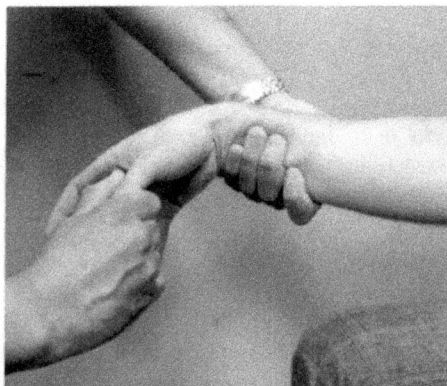

Figure 2.
Finkelstein's maneuver as described in 1930: the examiner pulls the thumb in ulnar deviation and longitudinal traction to exacerbate the symptoms of de Quervain's disease.

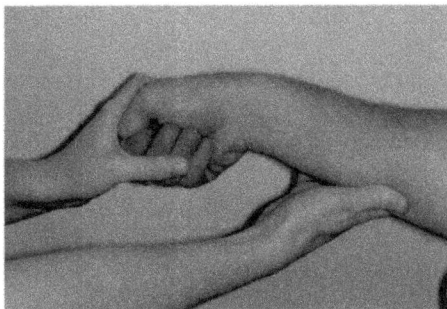

Figure 3.
Eichhoff's maneuver described in 1927, commonly confused with Finkelstein's test described in 1930.

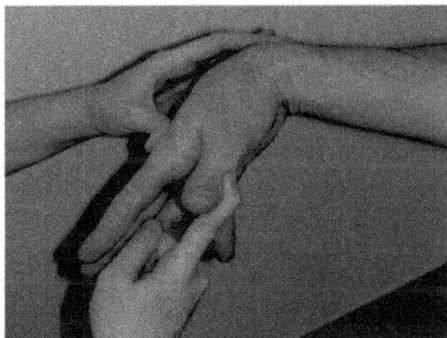

Figure 4.
WHAT test: active testing by shearing the tendons of the first extensor compartment against the palmar distal edge of the pulley.

5.2 Radiological diagnosis

5.2.1 Plain radiograph

Plain radiographs are nondiagnostic of the condition but may show nonspecific signs and can help exclude other causes of pain such as fracture, carpometacarpal arthritis, and osteomyelitis. Signs include [9]:

- Soft-tissue swelling over the radial styloid

- Focal abnormalities of the radial styloid including cortical erosion, sclerosis, or periosteal reaction

5.2.2 Ultrasound

Ultrasound is very often diagnostic. Findings include:

- Edematous tendon thickening of APL and EPB at the level of the radial styloid (compare with the contralateral side)

- Increased fluid within the first extensor tendon compartment tendon sheath

- Thickening of overlying retinaculum and the synovial sheath

- Peritendinous subcutaneous edema resulting in a hypoechoic halo sign

- Peritendinous subcutaneous hyperemia on Doppler imaging

It is important to assess for an intertendinous septum which can usually be identified if present. Ultrasound is often used to guide corticosteroid injections into the tendon compartment to treat the condition [10].

- Using B-mode ultrasound as standard, shear wave elastography (SWE) as diagnosis of de Quervain's tenosynovitis has 95% specificity and 85% sensitivity in diagnosing DQT.

- In addition, ultrasonic characteristics including a cutoff value of the extensor retinaculum for diagnosing DQT was 0.45 mm (sensitivity 96.3%, specificity 93.3%). Bony crests on the radial styloid were found in all cases of the presence of the intracompartmental septum [11].

5.2.3 MRI

MRI is very sensitive and specific and useful for detecting mild disease where ultrasound may be equivocal. The presence or absence of intertendinous septum can be assessed. Findings include:

- Tenosynovitis

  a. Increased fluid within tendon sheath (high T2, low-intermediate T1)

  b. Debris within sheath (intermediate T1 signal)

  c. Thickened edematous retinaculum

  d. Peritendinous subcutaneous edema

  e. Peritendinous subcutaneous contrast enhancement

- Tendinosis

  a. Tendon enlargement maximal at radial styloid and often greater at the medial aspect of the tendon

  b. Slightly increased intratendinous T1 and T2 signal compared to other tendons

  c. Striated appearance of tendons due to multiple enlarged slips

- Longitudinal tendon tear

  a. Linear high T2 signal due to fluid within the split

  b. More common in APL

5.2.4 Ultrasound-guided injections and prognosis in DQT

When comparing ultrasound and clinical characteristics of the operated and nonoperated wrists, it was found that patients with a high baseline visual analogue scale, with all positive clinical tests and with a persistent intracompartmental septum, had a significantly higher risk of failure following conservative treatment [12].

6. Evidence-based DQT therapy

A recent review article by Huisstede et al. [13] found (1) moderate evidence for the effect of corticosteroid injection on the very short term for DQT and (2) moderate evidence that a thumb splint as additive to a corticosteroid injection seems to be effective in the short term and midterm.

6.1 Ultrasound-guided partial release and simultaneous corticosteroid injection of DQT

One prospective study of 35 patients found that ultrasound-guided partial release and simultaneous corticosteroid injection using a 21-gauge needle was feasible in current practice, with minimal complications [14].

6.2 Corticosteroid injection (CSI)/CSI + splint for DQT

Prospectively randomized patients treated with either corticosteroid injection (CSI) alone were compared with CSI with immobilization [15]. Radial-sided wrist pain, first dorsal compartment tenderness, and positive Finkelstein test were used to define DQT. Pain score of 4 or higher on a visual analogue scale (VAS) was utilized for inclusion. Followed at 3 weeks and 6 months for further evaluation, resolution of symptoms and improvements in VAS and Disabilities of the Arm, Shoulder, and Hand (DASH) scores were assessed to evaluate treatment success. This small prospective controlled study (on 20 patients) found that immobilization of 3 weeks following injection increased costs, may hinder activities of daily living, and did not contribute to improved patient outcomes in this study.

Contrasting this, Awan et al. [16] found in a randomized controlled trial of 30 patients with established DQT that the use of therapeutic ultrasound and spica splint together is more effective than using therapeutic ultrasound alone in the conservative management over 6 months.

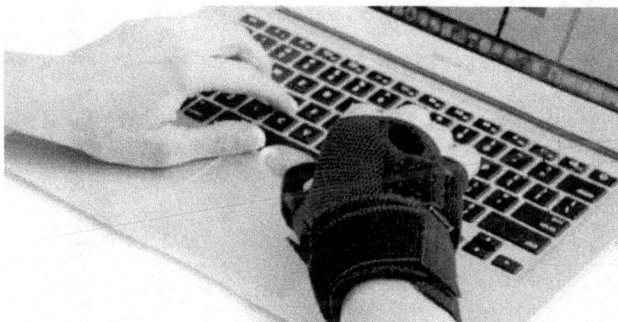

However, Cavaleri et al. [17] in an earlier review of six studies confirmed combined orthosis/corticosteroid injection approaches are more effective than either intervention alone. It was found that significantly more participants were treated successfully when combined orthosis/corticosteroid injection approaches were compared to (i) orthoses (RR 0.53, 95% CI 0.35–0.80) and (ii) injections alone (RR 0.76, 95% CI 0.64–0.89).

6.3 Surgical treatment for DQT

A follow up of 89 patients who underwent surgical treatment with the Le Viet technique with a follow-up of 9.5 years, were favorable, with total regression of functional impairment in 85% of cases and a satisfaction rate of 97.5%, with no cases of tendon dislocation, neuroma, or recurrence [18].

7. Conclusion

De Quervain's tenosynovitis (DQT) is one of the most common forms of stenosing tenosynovitis and is a common workplace injury. Diagnosis is usually clinical using either the Finkelstein's test, Eichhoff's test, and/or the wrist hyperflexion and abduction of the thumb (WHAT) test. If required, the single most useful and accurate investigation is a high-resolution ultrasound scan. This evidence-based review identified a clear approach to treatment of DQT including nonsurgical (therapeutic ultrasound with or without orthoses) and surgical approaches. However, we found that more high-quality RCTs are still needed to further stimulate evidence-based practice, especially related to work-related disorders.

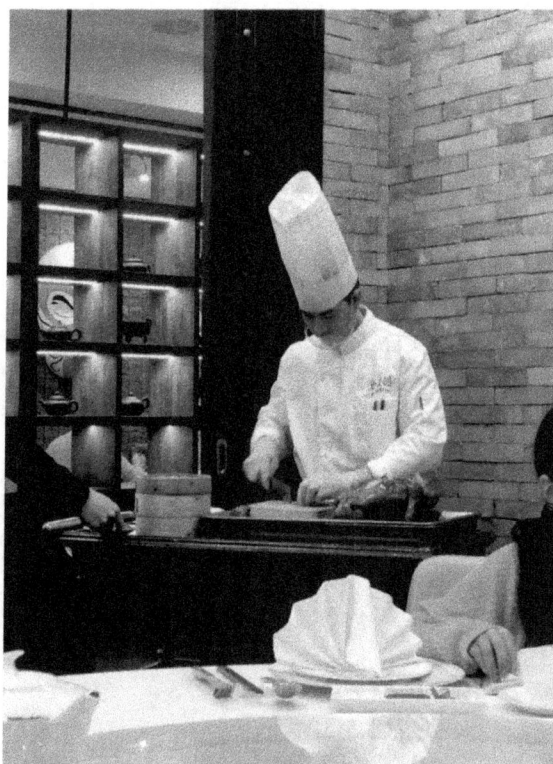

Author details

Jenson Mak[1,2,3,4*]

1 Rehabilitation Therapies Unit, Gosford Private Hospital, Australia

2 Healthy Ageing: Mind & Body, Sydney, Australia

3 University of Newcastle, Australia

4 John Walsh Centre for Rehabilitation, University of Sydney, Australia

*Address all correspondence to: jenson.mak@gmail.com

IntechOpen

References

[1] De Quervain F. Über eine Form von chronischer Tendovaginitis. Correspondenz-Blatt für Schweizer Aerzte, Basel; 1895;**25**:389-394

[2] Anderson BC. Office Orthopedics for Primary Care: Diagnosis and Treatment. 2nd ed. Philadelphia: WB Saunders; 1999

[3] Wolf JM, Sturdivant RX, Owens BD. Incidence of de Quervain's tenosynovitis in a young, active population. The Journal of Hand Surgery. 2009;**34**:112

[4] Stahl S, Vida D, Meisner C, Stahl AS, Schaller HE, Held M. Work related etiology of de Quervain's tenosynovitis: A case-control study with prospe tively collected data. BMC Musculoskeletal Disorders. 2015;**16**:126

[5] Clarke MT, Lyall HA, Grant JW, Matthewson MH. The histopathology of de Quervain's disease. The Journal of Hand Surgery: British and European. 1998;**23**:732

[6] Stahl S, Vida D, Meisner C, Lotter O, Rothenberger J, Schaller HE, et al. Systematic review and meta-analysis on the work-related cause of de Quervain tenosynovitis: A critical appraisal of its recognition as an occupational disease. Plastic and Reconstructive Surgery. 2013;**132**(6):1479-1491

[7] Huisstede BM, Coert JH, Fridén J, Hoogvliet P, European HANDGUIDE Group. Consensus on a multidisciplinary treatment guideline for de Quervain disease: Results from the European HANDGUIDE study. Physical Therapy. 2014;**94**(8):1095-1110

[8] Goubau JF, Goubau L, Van Tongel A, Van Hoonacker P, Kerckhove D, Berghs B. The wrist hyperflexion and abduction of the thumb (WHAT) test: A more specific and sensitive test to diagnose de Quervain tenosynovitis than the Eichhoff's test. The Journal of Hand Surgery, European Volume. 2014;**39**(3):286-292. DOI: 10.1177/1753193412475043. Epub 2013 Jan 22

[9] Lungu E, Dixon A, et al. De Quervain tenosynovitis. Radiopaedia. Available from: https://radiopaedia.org/articles/de-quervain-tenosynovitis [Accessed: September 2018]

[10] Turkay R, Inci E, Aydeniz B, Vural M. Shear wave elastography findings of de Quervain tenosynovitis. European Journal of Radiology. 2017;**95**:192-196

[11] Lee KH, Kang CN, Lee BG, Jung WS, Kim DY, Lee CH. Ultrasonographic evaluation of the first extensor compartment of the wrist in de Quervain's disease. Journal of Orthopaedic Science. 2014;**19**(1):49-54

[12] De Keating-Hart E, Touchais S, Kerjean Y, Ardouin L, Le Goff B. Presence of an intracompartmental septum detected by ultrasound is associated with the failure of ultrasound-guided steroid injection in de Quervain's syndrome. The Journal of Hand Surgery, European Volume. 2016;**41**(2):212-219

[13] Huisstede BM, Gladdines S, Randsdorp MS, Koes BW. Effectiveness of conservative, surgical, and postsurgical interventions for trigger finger, Dupuytren disease, and De Quervain disease: A systematic review. Archives of Physical Medicine and Rehabilitation. 2018;**99**(8):1635-1649.e21

[14] Lapègue F, André A, Pasquier Bernachot E, Akakpo EJ, Laumonerie P, Chiavassa-Gandois H, et al. US-guided percutaneous release of the first extensor tendon compartment using a 21-gauge needle in de Quervain's disease: A prospective study of 35

cases. European Radiology. 2018
Sep;**28**(9):3977-3985

[15] Ippolito JA, Hauser S, Patel J,
Vosbikian M, Ahmed I. Nonsurgical
treatment of De Quervain tenosynovitis:
A prospective randomized trial.
Hand (New York). 30 Jul 2018.
1558944718791187

[16] Awan WA, Babur MN, Masood
T. Effectiveness of therapeutic
ultrasound with or without thumb
spica splint in the management of De
Quervain's disease. Journal of Back
and Musculoskeletal Rehabilitation.
2017;**30**(4):691-697

[17] Cavaleri R, Schabrun SM, Te M,
Chipchase LS. Hand therapy versus
corticosteroid injections in the
treatment of de Quervain's disease:
A systematic review and meta-
analysis. Journal of Hand Therapy.
2016;**29**(1):3-11

[18] Garçon JJ, Charruau B, Marteau
E, Laulan J, Bacle G. Results of
surgical treatment of De Quervain's
tenosynovitis: 80 cases with a mean
follow-up of 9.5 years. Orthopaedics &
Traumatology, Surgery & Research. Oct
2018;**104**(6):893-896

Chapter 5

Lateral and Medial Epicondylitis: Definition, Diagnosis, Screening and Treatment Algorithms

Yusuf Erdem and Cagri Neyisci

Abstract

Medial/lateral epicondylitis is related to repetitive work activities which causes loss of labor. It sometimes becomes a chronic painful pathology. The main effect to protect the patients from such pathology should focus on avoiding repetitive patterns of work actually; however, it is not possible generally. Traditional treatment modalities such as physical therapies with the use of epicondylitis bands and intralesional steroid injections should be combined with newer modalities such as prolotherapy and prp injections in the treatment algorithm. In this chapter stages of the disease will be explained and those newer techniques and the mechanism of the healing would be detailed.

Keywords: elbow, tendonitis, forceful, rotation, forearm

1. Introduction

Work-related musculoskeletal disorder is an injury that occurs in the workplace or during the work due to sudden exertion or prolonged use of tendons, muscles, joints and nerves to physical factors such as repetitive movement, force or awkward positions. Shoulder disorders, lateral-medial epicondylitis, wrist tendinitis, and carpal tunnel syndromes in addition to other nonspecific strains, sprains are classified as common upper limb musculoskeletal disorders [1].

Epicondylitis is a common disorder of the arm that happens as a result of resisted use of the flexor and extensor muscles of the wrist. The men and women are affected equally, especially between fourth and fifth decades [2, 3]. Lateral epicondylitis, termed as *tennis elbow,* commonly occur after repeated activities of supination/pronation of the forearm while the elbow in extension, whereas medial epicondylitis, termed as *golfer's elbow*, mostly occur in athletes, tennis players, and workers whose jobs (e.g., carpentry) require similar movements [4–7]. Lateral epicondylitis is seen 5–10 times more than the medial epicondylitis [7, 8].

Treatment starts with conservative management including anti-inflammatory drug administration, physical therapy, rest, and steroid injections with variable long-term success.as soon as the diagnosis is confirmed, On the other hand the novel biological therapies which includes injection of platelet-rich plasma (PRP), collagen-producing tenocyte-like cells, various types of stem cells at the site of the tendon lesion, or prolotherapy are used as the developing treatment strategies [2, 9, 10]. Other treatment options include ultrasonographically guided tenotomy, extracorporeal shock-wave therapy, and iontophoresis and phonophoresis to obtain deep penetration of topical medications into the soft tissues [11]. Surgery is performed if there is no clinical response after 6–9 months of conservative treatment. Surgical techniques include open and arthroscopic approaches with dissection, release, and debridement of the degenerated and calcified tendons [12]. In our experience, we prefer a mini-open approach which allows a shorter recovery time and early postoperative mobilization therapy.

2. Elbow anatomy

2.1 Lateral elbow and epicondylitis

The extensor carpi radialis brevis, extensor digitorum communis, extensor carpi ulnaris, brachioradialis, extensor digiti minimi, supinator and extensor carpi radialis longus are called the wrist extensors, which allow the hand to move upward and extend. The wrist extensors form a strong conjoined tendon which is attached at the lateral epicondyle and lateral supracondylar ridge [13] (**Figure 1**). Repeated use of these tendons can cause microscopic tears and degeneration at the origin that can result forearm muscle weakness along with swelling and pain at the elbow. The ECRB forms the deep and anterior aspect of this common tendons and slides along capitellum's lateral edge during elbow extension and flexion. This contact and sliding may play a role in the pathophysiology of epicondylitis [4, 8, 14]. The essential lesion of lateral epicondylitis involves the ECRB mostly, followed by the extensor digitorum communis and to a lesser extent, other muscles and tendons of the lateral compartment. Capsular injury, thickening and tearing of the lateral ulnar collateral ligament (LUCL) and radial collateral ligament (RCL) have been also identified as another cause of lateral epicondylitis [14].

The lateral collateral ligament complex consists of the RCL, annular ligament, accessory lateral collateral ligament, and LUCL (**Figure 2**). Moreover, the LUCL runs along the lateral and posterior aspects of the radius to insert on the tubercle of the supinator crest of the ulna and disruption of which results in posterolateral rotatory instability of the elbow [14].

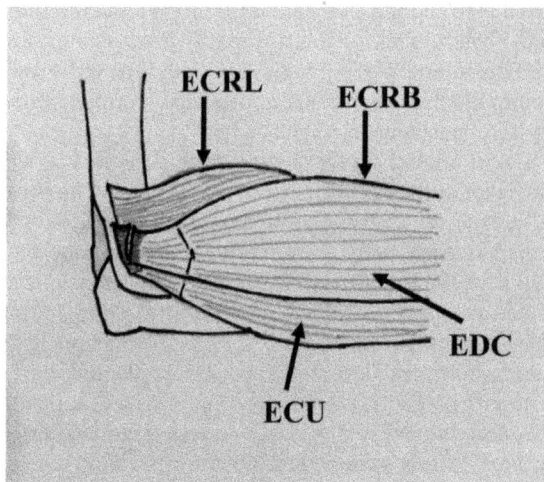

Figure 1.
Illustration shows the lateral elbow musculotendinous anatomy, close to the site of the tendon origin on the lateral epicondyle. ECRB = extensor carpi radialis brevis, CET = common extensor tendon, ECU = extensor carpi ulnaris, ECRL = extensor carpi radialis longus, and EDC = extensor digitorum communis [8].

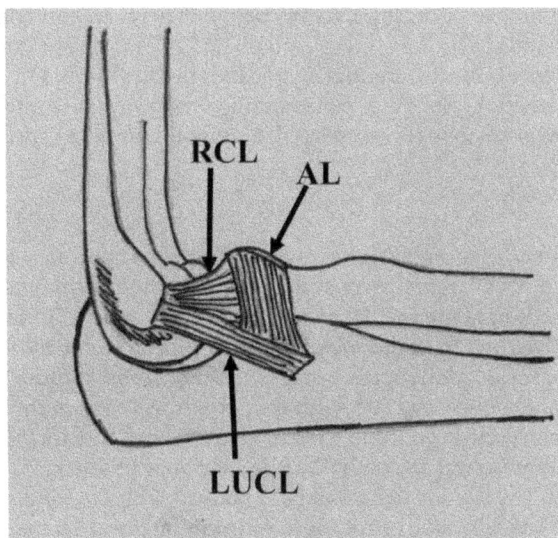

Figure 2.
Illustration shows the ligamentous anatomy of the lateral aspect of the elbow. AL = annular ligament, LUCL = lateral ulnar collateral ligament, and RCL = radial collateral ligament [8].

2.1.1 Etiology and pathophysiology

Lateral epicondylitis most commonly occurs between the ages of 30–50 years old. This pathology is caused by chronic stress to the forearm muscles with the repetitive activities of gripping and wrist extension. The most common movement that results with epicondylitis is radial deviation, extension of wrist, and forearm supination [15]. Many individuals develop lateral epicondylitis for no identifiable reason; however, poor mechanics or technique may be a reason in athletes.

As it is mentioned above, this condition is an overuse degenerative process of tendons of external carpi radialis brevis and extensor digitorum communis primarily. Beside clinical symptom of prolonged pain at the elbow, histological findings are granulation tissue, micro-rupture, an abundance of fibroblasts, vascular hyperplasia, unstructured collagen, and notably a lack of traditional inflammatory cells (macrophages, lymphocytes, neutrophils) within the tissue. In ultrasonographic evaluation calcifications, intrasubstance tears, thickening and heterogeneity of the common extensor tendon is mostly revealed [5, 15].

2.1.2 Physical examination

Provocative testing is done by performing the Cozen's test which is also known as resisted wrist extension test. During this test, the patient's elbow is stabilized in 90° of flexion by the examiner's thumb, while palpating over the patient's lateral epicondyle. The patient is then asked to make a fist, pronate the forearm, and radially deviate and extend the wrist while the manual resistance of the examiner. The test is considered positive if the test produces pain or reproductive of other symptoms in the area of the lateral epicondyle. Tenderness is usually seen over 5 mm. distal and anterior to the lateral epicondyle [15].

Mill's test is an alternative to Cozen's test, where the patient is asked to close the hand, with the wrist in dorsiflexion and the elbow extended. During the test, the wrist is forced into flexion, while palpating over the lateral epicondyle. The patient denies to do any motion, if he/she feels any pain on lateral epicondyle, and the test is considered positive [16].

On the other hand, the differential diagnosis is broad (**Table 1**), and imaging is often necessary when refractory or confounding symptoms are present. In a report, 5% reason of lateral epicondylitis is related with radial tunnel syndrome [17].

2.1.3 Diagnostic testing

Imaging of lateral epicondylitis not only confirms the clinical suspicion but also allows assessment of the injury severity and location. Multiple modalities such as magnetic resonance imaging (MRI), computed tomographic (CT) imaging, ultrasonography and EMG have been described following initial elbow radiography.

An initial x-ray evaluation should be taken in three views: anterior-posterior (AP), lateral, and lateral oblique view. The AP graphy is performed with the elbow fully extended, palm of the hand pointing upward (exorotation) and forearm supinated to display medial and lateral epicondyles as well as radiocapitellar and ulnotrochlear articular surfaces. The lateral view should be obtained with the hand is turned vertically, elbow in 90° of flexion, palm of the hand pointing toward patient and forearm in neutral position. Articulation between the distal humerus and proximal forearm is seen on these X-rays. Moreover the lateral oblique view is similar to the AP view, however the hand and forearm are fully externally rotated to obtain the views of the radiocapitellar joint, medial epicondyle, radioulnar joint and coronoid process.

X-rays can be helpful in evaluating bony structures' pathology, such as osteophyte formation secondary to arthritis, as well as calcifications that may be present in tendon or muscle tissues as a result of injury. Radiographic evaluations show normal results in most cases, and are mainly useful for ruling out other abnormalities such as arthrosis, osteochondritis dissecans and intra-articular free bodies. When X-ray is inconclusive, further studies such as MRI, ultrasound, or CT scan may be ordered.

Sonography is an inexpensive, accessible and radiation-free test. Moreover high-frequency probes has an advantages of improved resolution, allowing application to extraarticular soft tissues for which it is increasingly used as an alternative to MRI [18]. Additionally, dynamic imaging can be performed in flexion/extension, supination/pronation, or under valgus/varus stress. Dynamic sonography is also an ideal method of image-guided intervention and can be used to provide real-time guidance of injections of local anesthetic, steroids, or platelet-rich plasma. However, its value is debatable because it is examiner-dependent.

In many cases MRI can be useful in evaluating the soft tissues for tears, fluid, inflammation, or other changes within the joint or surrounding tissues. It is a great tool to evaluate soft tissue damage due to chronic overuse injuries of the elbow. However the bony cortex is not as well evaluated at MR imaging compared with CT, but the ability to detect subtle signal intensity changes in the marrow and periosteal soft tissues increases sensitivity to early stress changes in bone. Patients positioning

Posterolateral rotatory instability, LUCL injury
Osteochondritis dissecans of the capitellum
Occult fracture
Radial tunnel syndrome
Osteoarthrosis

Table 1.
Differential diagnosis of lateral elbow pain.

can be either prone or supine, with the arm held at the side in anatomical position. Initial evaluation includes the assessment of the radiocapitellar, ulnohumeral and radioulnar articulations of the elbow. The following examination steps are tendons, muscles, ligaments, and the three major nerves of the elbow [19, 20].

CT imaging is particularly useful in demonstrating intraarticular extension of fractures, the distribution of small fracture fragments within and adjacent to the joint space, as well as any associated bony malalignment. CT can also be useful in evaluating chronic pain following injury and can readily identify abnormal ossifications or calcifications which can be seen as a sequela of trauma, including osteochondral bodies, heterotopic ossification, or myositis ossificans. Intraarticular contrast material can be injected for improved visualization of joint bodies and cartilage. Osseous manifestations of secondary degenerative change are also well evaluated with CT. Less often, CT arthrography is performed for evaluation of ligamentous integrity in patients with contraindications to MR imaging [18].

Aside from imaging, many elbow pain cases will require an electromyography/nerve conduction study to investigate the function of forearm muscle in healthy and diseased. This test consists of two parts, and utilizes needle EMG to test the muscles in the extremity. It may be helpful in nerve compressive processes. The needle EMG may reveal the differentiation between denervation versus nerve injury or compression [21]. However future diagnosing studies are essential for this test.

In case of significant swelling or fever, blood work should be indicated whether the reason is systemic inflammation or not. This would help direct the treatment toward a systemic, rheumatologic, or infectious etiology [21, 22].

2.2 Medial elbow and epicondylitis

The medial epicondyle is the common origin of the flexor and pronator muscles of the forearm. Five muscles (flexor carpi radialis, palmaris longus, flexor carpi ulnaris, flexor digitorum superficialis and pronator teres) share the same origin and form the conjoined flexor tendons (**Figure 3**) [7]. The MCL, or known as ulnar collateral ligament, is formed by anterior, posterior, and oblique bands, which creates a triangular shape along the medial aspect of the elbow, deep to the pronator mass

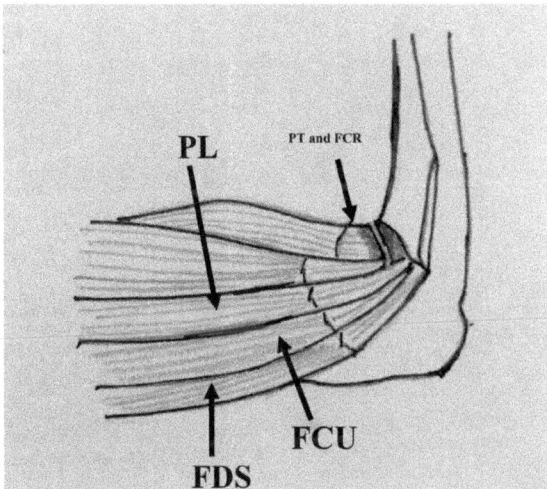

Figure 3.
Illustration shows the medial elbow musculotendinous anatomy. FCU = flexor carpi ulnaris, FCR = flexor carpi radialis, FDS = flexor digitorum superficialis, PT = pronator teres, and PL = palmaris longus [8].

(**Figure 4**). MCL injury, specifically anterior band injury, is included in the differential diagnosis of medial elbow pain, and therefore the MCL must be evaluated. The MCL is also prone to concurrent injury with me- dial epicondylitis.

Medial epicondylitis is a tendinopathy of conjoined tendon due to overload or overuse. This pathology is also called golfer's elbow which mostly develops as a result of high energy valgus forces in athletes. However 90% of cases are not sports-related.

2.2.1 Physical examination

Patients with medial epicondylitis typically present with medial elbow pain, which often develops due to repetitive elbow use, gripping, or valgus stress. The pain is worse with forearm motion, hand gripping and throwing. It usually resolves with cessation of activity [4, 7, 23]. On physical examination, there may be tenderness, swelling, erythema or warmth. The tenderness is elicited by palpation over the 5–10 mm distal and anterior to the medial epicondyle [4].

Medial epicondylitis test involves an active and passive component where the pain is exacerbated by resisted wrist flexion and forearm pronation at an angle of 90° [7]. Test is positive when the patient endorses pain with this maneuver. Due to similar symptoms and associated valgus forces, C6–C7 radiculopathies, cubital tunnel syndrome, ulnar neuritis, anterior interosseous nerve entrapment, tardy ulnar palsy and MCL instability, as well as other causes of medial elbow pain (capsulitis, arthrofibrosis, loose bodies, or medial epicondyle avulsion fracture) should be considered in the differential diagnosis (**Table 2**). The Tinel sign (distal pain and tingling during direct compression of the nerve at the elbow) should be used to evaluate for ulnar neuropathy, and the ulnar collateral ligament should be stressed especially in athletes [23]. The elbow valgus stress test is used to assess the integrity of the medial collateral ligament by palpating the medial joint line and stabilizing the distal humerus in 20 degrees of elbow flexion, [23]. The tests are considered positive if the patient experiences pain or excessive laxity along the MCL compared to the contralateral side.

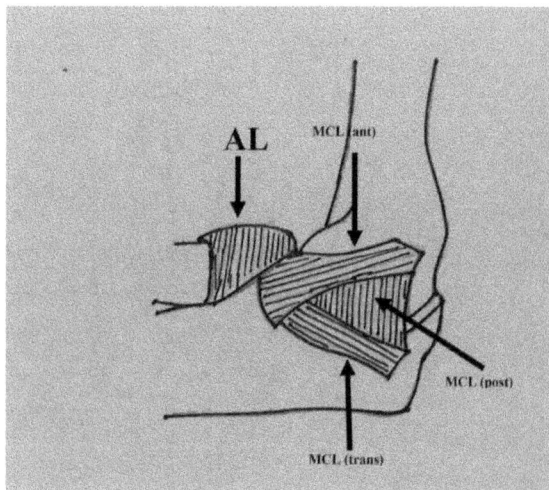

Figure 4.
Picture shows the ligamentous anatomy of the medial aspect of the elbow. AL = annular ligament, ant = anterior band, and post = posterior band [8].

MCL İnjury
Little League Elbow
Osteochondritis dissecans (OCD)
Ulnar neuropathy (ulnar neuritis, entrapment)
Flexor-pronator strain
Occult fracture

Table 2.
Differential diagnosis of medial elbow pain.

2.2.2 Etiology and pathophysiology

Medial epicondylitis is generally considered to start as a microtear due to chronic stress which is related with repetitive concentric or eccentric loading of the wrist flexors and pronator teres, resulting angiofibroblastic changes. Angiofibroblastic changes include mucoid degeneration of the tendinous origin and formation of reactive granulation tissue [24]. As a result focal necrosis or calcification can occur with decreasing collagen strength, scar tissue formation, and thickening of the tendons. Though it was thought that the pronator teres and flexor carpi radialis were most commonly affected, the studies suggest that all muscles except palmaris longus are affected equally [20].

Though the conservative treatment is a common intervention for the treatment, surgical treatment is applied to remove the pathologic tissues around these origins (the common flexor origin) to eliminate pain generators and decompression to promote tissue regeneration in chronic pathology.

2.2.3 Diagnostic testing

As in lateral epicondylitis, imaging is not always essential in the initial evaluation of medial epicondylitis. Radiographs are most useful to rule out other causes of elbow pain and usually normal in this pathology. Especially, in children where the diagnosis is uncertain, comparison to the unaffected arm may be necessary.

Sonography is also a quick, easy and cost-effective modality to evaluate tendon pathology and distinguish from other etiologies. Moreover dynamic evaluation can be done in areas of chronic degeneration.

MRI is the ideal diagnostic imaging modality in medial epicondylitis and rule out other possible causes of elbow pain like MCL strain, osteochondritis dissecans, or other soft tissue injuries.

Computed tomography, electromyogram and bone scan may be useful in refractory cases to rule out other etiologies as well [23].

2.2.4 Treatment

Once the diagnosis is clear, offending activities including decreasing the volume, frequency, or intensity should be cascaded. Beside, patients may respond to non-steroidal anti-inflammatory drugs and acetaminophen as an initial step. Also topical nitroglycerin patches have proven helpful in the treatment of tendinopathies. Most cases of epicondylitis are managed conservatively. Though medial epicondylitis is less common compared to lateral epicondylitis, the treatment is more difficult.

The primary goal of the first step of treatment includes pain and inflammation relief. Modification of life style is important. Physical therapy takes a great role for the management of treatment simultaneously. Multiple physical therapy modalities including dry needling, etracorporeal shock wave therapy, iontophoresis, electrical stimulation and ultrasonography takes great role to overcome this pathology [25–28]. Theoretically, eccentric strengthening efficiently induces hypertrophy of the musculotendinous unit and increases it tensile strength, thereby reducing strain of the tendon. Therapy was more effective than rest and restriction of activities.

Counterforce bracing (forearm bands) inhibits full muscular expansion and decreases the force on the muscular tissue proximal to the brace. Night splinting with a cock up wrist splint and elbow kinesio taping may be helpful. In case of non-compliance or when these treatment modalities are not available injections are used. Currently corticosteroids (especially betamethasone sodium phosphate and dipropionate) and local anesthetic mixture is the most common, however recent studies have shown a new group of injectable substances such as botulinum toxin, autologous blood, platelet-rich plasma, hyaluronic acid and prolotherapy are being utilized [29]. Recent studies have shown that Visual Analog Scale (VAS) pain scores and functional scores during the first 2–6 weeks (acute period) have improved after the injections mentioned above [2]. However the dose and frequency of the corticosteroids or others is still controversial. Moreover the corticosteroid injection may result with local skin atrophy, depigmentation and muscle wasting [2].

Botulinum toxin A have been shown as an off-label treatment and have some literature support in refractory cases. It has also has the ability to cause a partial paralysis of the wrist flexors and extensors and allow the pathologic tissue to heal while avoiding micro trauma to the tendon. In a study, 60 patients who received a blinded injection of botulinum toxin or placebo have been evaluated with results of significant lower VAS pain scores at 4 and 12 weeks in the botulinum toxin group. On the other hand the major adverse effect seen with botulinum toxin injection is finger and wrist extensor weakness [30].

Autologous blood injection has been described by Edwards and Calandruccio [31]. Autologous platelet-rich plasma (PRP) have been shown to reduce pain and improve function in refractory epicondylitis [31]. Mishra and Pavelko reported significantly better VAS and functional scores at 8-week period compared to placebo [32]. In conclusion, the effect of remaining injection modalities, which are known as PRP and autologous whole blood, are about the chronic cases with a persistent efficacy during long term follow up. At the end hyaluronic acid and prolotherapy injections have also been studied for epicondylitis have been found to be effective in refractory cases however the mechanism is not well known [33, 34].

Surgical indications for medial and lateral epicondylitis include persistent pain and weakness of the forearm that persists after a period of at least 6 months of conservative care, however it is usually not needed. These surgeries involve release of the common flexor and extensor tendon at the epicondyle and debridement of pathologic tissue. The mini-open muscle resection involves removal of degenerative tissue of the flexor carpi radialis. Fascial elevation and tendon origin resection is another available technique [34]. The prognosis for recovery is very good with relief of pain, but often results in weakness of the forearm musculature [33].

3. Discussion

Medial and lateral epicondylitis is a chronic inflammation disease which results in loss of labor. Moreover these pathologies are related with other upper extremity abnormalities most of which are accompanied with cervical disc pathologies. Physician should be aware of other conditions which led to or mimics epicondylitis.

The patients' social status and job should be questioned at first intervention, thus the treatment varies depending on the situation. If a pure epicondylitis is diagnosed the treatment algorithm is defined above beginning conservatively at first to surgery at last. The aim of the treatment is directed to return to activity as well.

Author details

Yusuf Erdem[1*] and Cagri Neyisci[2]

1 Gulhane Training and Research Hospital, Ankara, Turkey

2 Gulhane Training and Research Hospital, Department of Orthopaedic Surgey, Ankara, Turkey

*Address all correspondence to: yerdem81@gmail.com

IntechOpen

References

[1] Bepko J, Mansalis K. Common occupational disorders: Asthma, COPD, dermatitis, and musculoskeletal disorders. American Family Physician. 2016;**93**(12):1000-1006

[2] Tarpada SP, Morris MT, Lian J, Rashidi S. Current advances in the treatment of medial and lateral epicondylitis. Journal of Orthopaedics. 2018;**15**(1):107-110

[3] Shiri R, Viikari-Juntura E, Varonen H, Heliövaara M. Prevalence and determinants of lateral and medial epicondylitis: A population study. American Journal of Epidemiology. 2006;**164**(11):1065-1074

[4] Bernard FM, Regan WD. Elbow and forearm. In: DeLee JC, editor. DeLee and Drez's Orthopaedic Sports Medicine. 2nd ed. Philadelphia, PA: Saunders; 2003

[5] Nirschl RP, Pettrone FA. Lateral and medial epicondylitis. In: Morrey BF, editor. Master Techniques in Orthopedic Surgery: The Elbow. New York, NY: Raven; 1994. pp. 537-552

[6] Coonrad RW, Hooper WR. Tennis elbow: Its course, natural history, conservative and surgical management. The Journal of Bone and Joint Surgery. American Volume. 1973;**55**:1177-1182

[7] Ciccotti MC, Schwartz MA, Ciccotti MG. Diagnosis and treatment of medial epicondylitis of the elbow. Clinics in Sports Medicine. 2004;**23**:693-705

[8] Walz DM, Newman JS, Konin GP, Ross G. Epicondylitis: Pathogenesis, imaging, and treatment. RadioGraphics. 2010;**30**(1):167-184

[9] Ikpe S, Lesniak B. Biologics and cell-based treatments for upper extremity injuries. Operative Techniques in Orthopaedics. 2016;**26**(3):177-181

[10] Connell D, Datir A, Alyas F, Curtis M. Treatment of lateral epicondylitis using skin-derived tenocyte-like cells. British Journal of Sports Medicine. 2009;**43**(4):293-298

[11] Faro F, Wolf JM. Lateral epicondylitis: Review and current concepts. The Journal of Hand Surgery. 2007;**32**:1271-1279

[12] Cohen MS, Romeo AA, Hennigan SP, Gordon M. Lateral epicondylitis: Anatomic relationship of the extensor tendon origins and implications for arthroscopic treatment. Journal of Shoulder and Elbow Surgery. 2008;**17**:954-960

[13] Blease S, Stoller DW, Safran MR, Li AE, Fritz RC. The elbow. In: Stoller DW, editor. Magnetic Resonance Imaging in Orthopaedics and Sports Medicine. 3rd ed. Philadelphia, PA: Lippincott, Williams & Wilkins; 2007. pp. 1463-1626

[14] Bunata RE, Brown DS, Capelo R. Anatomic factors related to the cause of tennis elbow. The Journal of Bone and Joint Surgery. American Volume. 2007;**89**:1955-1963

[15] Smidt N, Lewis M, Van Der Windt DA, Hay EM, Bouter LM, Croft P. Lateral epicondylitis in general practice: Course and prognostic indicators of outcome. The Journal of Rheumatology. 2006;**33**(10):2053-2059

[16] Filho M, Cotovelo GR. In: Barros Filho TEP, Lech O, editors. Exame Físico em Ortopedia. São Paulo: Sarvier; 2001. pp. 138-156

[17] Ferdinand BD, Rosenberg ZS, Schweitzer ME, et al. MR imaging features of radial tunnel syndrome: Initial experience. Radiology. 2006;**240**:161-168

[18] Potter HG. Imaging of posttraumatic and soft tissue dysfunction of the elbow. Clinical Orthopaedics. 2000;**370**:9-18

[19] Hoffman AD, Graviss ER. Imaging of the pediatric elbow. In: The Elbow and its Disorders. Philadephia, PA: Saunders; 2000. pp. 155-163

[20] Srinath CS, Srihari S, Miriam B. Magnetic resonance imaging of the elbow: A structured approach. Sports Health. 2013;**5**(1):34-49

[21] Braddom RL, Chan L, Harrast MA, Kowalske KJ, Matthews DJ, Ragnarsson KT, et al. Physical Medicine and Rehabilitation. 4th ed. Philadelphia: Saunders; pp. 825-838

[22] Bonica JJ. In: Fishman S, Ballantyne J, Rathmell JP, editors. Bonica's Management of Pain. Philadelphia: Lippincott Williams & Wilkins; 2010. pp. 1034-1028

[23] Han SH, Lee JK, Kim HJ, Lee SH, Kim JW, Kim TS. The result of surgical treatment of medial epicondylitis: Analysis with more than a 5-year follow-up. Journal of Shoulder and Elbow Surgery. 2016;**25**(10):1704-1709

[24] Goran R, Violeta Vm Mihaela M, Rodina N, Tzvetanka P, Francesco P, Annamaria I. Ultrasound assessment of the elbow. Medical Ultrasonography. 2012;**14**(2):141-146

[25] Labelle H, Guibert R. "Efficacy of Diclofenac in lateral epicondylitis of the elbow also treated with immobilization:" The University of Montreal Orthopaedic Reseach

Group. Archives of Family Medicine. 1997;**6**:257-262

[26] Burnham R, Gregg R, Healy P, Steadward R. The effectiveness of topical Diclofenac for lateral epicondylitis. Clinical Journal of Sport Medicine. 1998;**8**:78-81

[27] Bisset L, Paungmali A, Vincenzino B, Beller E. A systematic review and meta analysis of clinical trials on physical interventions for lateral epicondylalgia. British Journal of Sports Medicine. 2005;**39**:411-422

[28] Pettrone FA, McCall BR. Extracorporeal shock wave therapy without local anesthesia for chronic lateral epicondylitis. The Journal of Bone and Joint Surgery. American Volume. 2005;**87**:1297-1304

[29] Groppel JL, Nirschl RP. A mechanical and electromyographical analysis of the effects of various joint counterforce braces on the tennis player. The American Journal of Sports Medicine. 1986;**14**:195-200

[30] Sm W, Hui AC, Tong PY, Poon DW, Yu E, Wong LK. Treatment of lateral epicondylitis with botulinum toxin: A randomized, double-blind, placebo-controlled trail. Annals of Internal Medicine. 2005;**143**(1):793-797

[31] Edwards SG, Calandruccio JH. Autologous blood injections for refractory lateral epicondylitis. The Journal of Hand Surgery. 2003 Mar;**28**(2):272-278

[32] Mishra A, Pavelko T. Treatment of chronic elbow tendinosis with buffered platelet-rich plasma. The American Journal of Sports Medicine. 2006;**34**:1774-1778

[33] Degen RM, Cancienne JM, Camp CL, Altchek DW, Dines JS, Werner BC. Patient-related risk factors for

requiring surgical intervention
following a failed injection for the
treatment of medial and lateral
epicondylitis. The Physician and
Sportsmedicine. 2017;**45**(4):433-437

[34] Raeissadat SA, Ranyegani SM,
Hassanabadi H, Rahimi R, Sedighipour
L, Rostami K. Is platelet-rich plasma
superior to whole blood in the
management of chronic tennis elbow:
One year randomized clinical trial.
BMC Sports Science, Medicine and
Rehabilitation. 2014;**6**(1):12